D0829805

100 Questions & Answers About Your Child's Schizophrenia

Josiane Cobert, MD

Child and Adolescent Psychiatrist
North Shore University Hospital
Elizabeth, NJ

JONES AND BARTLETT PUBLISHERS
Sudbury, Massachusetts
BOSTON   TORONTO   LONDON   SINGAPORE

World Headquarters
Jones and Bartlett
Publishers
40 Tall Pine Drive
Sudbury, MA 01776
978-443-5000
info@jbpub.com
www.jbpub.com

Jones and Bartlett
Publishers Canada
6339 Ormindale Way
Mississauga, Ontario L5V 1J2
Canada

Jones and Bartlett
Publishers International
Barb House, Barb Mews
London W6 7PA
United Kingdom

Jones and Bartlett's books and products are available through most bookstores and online book-sellers. To contact Jones and Bartlett Publishers directly, call 800-832-0034, fax 978-443-8000, or visit our website, www.jbpub.com.

Substantial discounts on bulk quantities of Jones and Bartlett's publications are available to corpo-rations, professional associations, and other qualified organizations. For details and specific dis-count information, contact the special sales department at Jones and Bartlett via the above contact information or send an email to specialsales@jbpub.com.

Copyright © 2010 by Jones and Bartlett Publishers, LLC

All rights reserved. No part of the material protected by this copyright may be reproduced or utilized in any form, electronic or mechanical, including photocopying, recording, or by any information storage and retrieval system, without written permission from the copyright owner.

The authors, editor, and publisher have made every effort to provide accurate information. However, they are not responsible for errors, omissions, or for any outcomes related to the use of the contents of this book and take no responsibility for the use of the products and procedures described. Treat-ments and side effects described in this book may not be applicable to all people; likewise, some people may require a dose or experience a side effect that is not described herein. Drugs and medical devices are discussed that may have limited availability controlled by the Food and Drug Adminis-tration (FDA) for use only in a research study or clinical trial. Research, clinical practice, and gov-ernment regulations often change the accepted standard in this field. When consideration is being given to use of any drug in the clinical setting, the health care provider or reader is responsible for determining FDA status of the drug, reading the package insert, and reviewing prescribing information for the most up-to-date recommendations on dose, precautions, and contraindications, and determining the appropriate usage for the product. This is especially important in the case of drugs that are new or seldom used.

Production Credits
Senior Acquisitions Editor: Alison Hankey
Editorial Assistant: Sara Cameron
Associate Production Editor: Leah Corrigan
Senior Marketing Manager: Barb Bartoszek
Manufacturing and Inventory Supervisor: Amy Bacus
Composition: Glyph International
Cover Design: Carolyn Downer
Cover Images: © Pete Saloutos/ShutterStock, Inc., © LiquidLibrary, © iofoto/ShutterStock, Inc.
Printing and Binding: Malloy, Inc.
Cover Printing: Malloy, Inc.

Library of Congress Cataloging-in-Publication Data
Cobert, Josiane.
    100 questions & answers about your child's schizophrenia / Josiane Cobert.
        p. cm.
    Includes index.
    ISBN 978-0-7637-7808-8 (alk. paper)
    1. Schizophrenia in children--Miscellanea. 2. Schizophrenia--Popular works.
    I. Title. II. Title: One hundred questions and answers about your child's schizophrenia.
    RJ506.S3C63 2010
        618.92'898—dc22
    6048   2009031501

Printed in the United States of America
13 12 11 10 09   10 9 8 7 6 5 4 3 2 1

To my children, Emilie and Julien.

Contents

Contents

The word *schizophrenia* may bring to mind the real life stories of John Nash or Andrea Yates, whose lives have been reported in books and movies. John Nash, a mathematician who won the Nobel Prize, became very sick with a schizophrenic disorder in young adulthood, which ended his academic career. Yates, a mother of five, was suffering from depression and schizophrenia. She drowned her young children to "save them from the devil" and is now in prison.

Roughly 1% of the world's population has schizophrenia, and most remain largely disabled throughout adulthood. The disease usually presents in early adult life, so psychiatrists have been cautious about making this diagnosis in children and adolescents. Because of this hesitance, there is confusion about the disease in children. This book will try to clarify some of the problems.

PART ONE

The Basics

What is "Childhood Schizophrenia" (also called
Child Onset Schizophrenia [COS])?

What is the difference between thought disorder,
psychosis (psychotic thinking), schizophrenic-like
psychosis, and schizophrenia?

Is my child insane?

More . . .

1. What is "Childhood Schizophrenia" (also called Child Onset Schizophrenia or COS)?

Schizophrenia

Any of a group of psychotic disorders usually characterized by withdrawal from reality, illogical patterns of thinking, delusions, and hallucinations.

DSM-IV

The Diagnostic and Statistical Manual developed by leading clinical psychiatrists in the United States for the systematic evaluation of psychiatric patients and assigning diagnoses to groups of symptoms.

Psychotic

People are considered psychotic if they have lost touch with reality, have delusions (i.e., false beliefs), and hallucinations.

Negative symptoms

Those characteristics of psychiatric illness that present as withdrawn behavior, an expressionless face, a lack of initiative, a lack of interest, and slow speech.

Positive symptoms

Considered the active symptoms of hallucinations and delusions of schizophrenia.

The definition of this disease has been the object of considerable debate over the years. What is clear is that it is a chronic, severe mental illness that can be very debilitating. Making the diagnosis is difficult enough, but there was confusion about whether childhood **schizophrenia** is different from adult schizophrenia or if it is a continuum of the same disease. Child Schizophrenia is seen as an early manifestation of schizophrenia as it is recognized in adults. There is now ample evidence that the abnormalities are similar in childhood and adult schizophrenia and to suggest that it is a continuum along the lifetime of the individual.

The current diagnostic criteria for schizophrenia are described in the **DSM-IV**-TR (Diagnostic and Statistical Manual of Mental Disorders, fourth edition, Text revision from the American Psychiatric Association, 2000). Created by psychiatrists and published by the American Psychiatric Association, the DSM-IV sets the standards and definitions for mental disorders. It is used extensively in the United States and in many other parts of the world.

The disorder is defined by **psychotic** symptoms (psychosis), deficits in social functioning and a duration of at least 6 months.

The active psychotic symptoms include positive or **negative symptoms**.

Positive symptoms are:

- **Delusions** (a false belief based on faulty judgment about one's environment)

- **Hallucinations** (the perception of something such as a sound or visual image that is not actually present other than in the mind)
- **Disorganizational Syndrome** with disorganized speech (incoherent, nonlogical, derailed speech, not getting to the point, vague) and grossly disorganized or **catatonic behavior** (extreme loss of motor skills or constant hyperactivity)

Negative symptoms include:

- Flat affect (not showing emotions)
- Alogia (poverty of speech)
- Avolition (lack of initiative or motivation)

If delusions are bizarre, or if the auditory hallucination consists of a voice running a commentary about the person's thoughts or behavior or if there are two or more voices having a conversation with each other, then only one active phase symptom is necessary for the diagnosis.

Social or occupational dysfunction is usually present and is defined as the failure to achieve the expected level of self-care, interpersonal, academic, or occupational achievement.

The 6-month period must include at least 1 month of the active phase symptoms and may include periods of **prodromal** (initial or early symptoms before the active phase) or **residual** (late or remaining after the active phase) symptoms. In these phases, the signs of the disturbance may be seen only by negative symptoms or symptoms that are present in a mild or attenuated form like odd beliefs or unusual perceptual experiences.

The Basics

Delusions
A false belief based on faulty judgment about one's environment.

Hallucinations
Experiencing something from any of the five senses that is not occurring in reality.

Disorganizational Syndrome
A set of symptoms related to general disorganization (speech and/or behavioral disorganization).

Catatonic behavior
Behavior characterized by muscular tightness or rigidity and lack of response to the environment.

Prodromal
An early or premonitory symptom of a disease.

Residual
Having some non-specific symptoms (usually negative symptoms), but no longer active psychotic ones.

The disorder cannot be diagnosed if the patient has certain other different psychiatric problems (such as schizoaffective or mood disorder with psychotic features), nor can it result from the direct effects of drugs (legal or illicit), medications, or a medical condition.

Schizoaffective

Having both prominent symptoms of schizophrenia and depression and/or mania that overlap with the schizophrenia-like symptoms.

Substance abuse

The continued use of alcohol and or other drugs despite negative consequences like social, legal, and relational problems.

The disorder cannot be diagnosed if the patient has certain other different psychiatric problems (such as **schizoaffective** or mood disorder with psychotic features), nor can it result from the direct effects of drugs (legal or illicit), medications, or a medical condition.

If there is a history of autistic disorder or another major developmental disorder, then the additional diagnosis of schizophrenia is made only if delusions or hallucinations are also present for at least 1 month (or less if successfully treated).

Many problems arise in applying adult criteria to children and adolescents. For example:

- Disorganized speech and behavior are common in nonpsychotic children and may result in making the diagnosis of schizophrenia when it is not the case.
- Adolescents who have schizophrenia may have a history of **substance abuse** so the diagnosis of schizophrenia may be overlooked.
- The concept of psychosis is very problematic in children. Children's conceptions of reality change over the course of normal development and many children believe in fantasy figures for a period of time, which is not psychosis or schizophrenia.
- The presence together (**comorbidity**) in the same child of schizophrenia and autism makes the diagnosis of schizophrenia difficult. Because of this, there are false-positives (erroneously making the diagnosis) and false-negatives (erroneously missing the diagnosis).
- The presence of mental retardation or other developmental disorders makes it difficult to assess psychotic thinking in children.

- If a child does not talk, psychosis or any thought disorder is very difficult to evaluate.

This shows how complex it is to make the diagnosis of schizophrenia in children, especially in very young ones. The parent and the physician must incorporate a long term developmental point of view when thinking about psychosis in children. The situation is not static, changes occur and reevaluations must be done periodically.

From a teacher:

*Thomas is 6 years old. He could not sit still in the classroom, did not follow any directions from me. When asked to do something, he had severe temper tantrums. If a peer answered for him, he became aggressive. He has thrown books around the room, turned over chairs. When I asked him why he did those things he told me that a voice in his head told him to do that and he was following orders. Every reaction seemed out of proportion. He even bit me once when I reprimanded him. He was disorganized, forgetful. I thought that he had Attention Deficit Hyperactivity Disorder (**ADHD**) but his mother told me that the doctor felt he was psychotic and that it might be the beginning of schizophrenia. His mother told me that her own brother had been diagnosed with schizophrenia in the past. Thomas is staying in the hospital for his treatment and is doing better.*

2. What is the difference between thought disorder, psychosis (psychotic thinking), schizophrenic-like psychosis, and schizophrenia?

All these terms are very confusing and we will try to define them:

Comorbidity

Coexistence of two or more disorders in the same individual.

The Basics

ADHD

A disorder characterized by short attention span, hyperactivity, and impulsivity.

Table 1   Terminology

Terms	Definition	Disorders
Thought Disorder	A state in which there is disordered speech which is felt to reflect disordered and abnormal thought processes and thinking.	A thought disorder is not a disease in and of itself but rather a description of the patient's state. It may be caused by many things including psychosis and schizophrenia but also from stress, drugs, and many other causes (i.e., neurological diseases, intoxication, endocrine problems, developmental disorders).
Psychosis Psychotic thought process Psychotic thought disorder Psychotic thinking Psychotic symptoms (All of these terms are used synonymously)	A mental state or symptoms described as involving a "loss of contact with reality." People suffering from psychosis are said to be psychotic. People experiencing psychosis may report hallucinations or delusional beliefs, and may exhibit personality changes and disorganized thinking.	Psychosis can be a symptom of mental illness, but it is not a mental illness in its own right. Psychosis can be seen in many other diseases or situations.
Schizophrenia	A disease which must meet the DSM IV criteria (see question 1).	It is a chronic mental illness or disease.
Schizotypal	Characterized as needing social isolation and with odd behavior and thinking and often unconventional beliefs.	Schizotypal personality disorder.
Very early onset schizophrenia (VEOS)	Schizophrenia that develops before the age of 13 years old.	
Early onset schizophrenia (EOS)	Schizophrenia that develops after the age of 13 and before 18 years.	
Schizophrenic-like psychosis	Schizophrenic-like psychosis is a symptom and is a psychosis that looks like the psychosis present in schizophrenia but not due to schizophrenia.	May be due to a mood disorder or medical problems.

Table 1 (*Continued*)

Terms	Definition	Disorders
Schizophreniform disorder	A disorder very similar to schizophrenia but which has been lasting for more than 1 month and less than 6 months.	
Psychotic disorders	A disease that is characterized by psychotic thought processes.	The DSM-IV-TR lists nine formal psychotic disorders, but many other disorders may have psychotic symptoms. The formal psychotic disorders are: 1. Schizophrenia 2. Schizoaffective disorder 3. Schizophreniform disorder 4. Brief psychotic disorder 5. Delusional disorder 6. Shared psychotic disorder (Folie à deux) 7. Substance induced psychosis 8. Psychosis due to a general medical condition 9. Psychosis—Not otherwise specified

The Basics

Earlier theories (since Bleuler, 1951) described thought disorder as the hallmark of schizophrenia. In the late 1970s, it was demonstrated that thought disorder does not occur exclusively in schizophrenia but occurs in other mental disorders also. Some differentiation has been made and three aspects of psychotic thinking in children are described.

In the late 1970s, it was demonstrated that thought disorder does not occur exclusively in schizophrenia but occurs in other mental disorders also.

- A formal thought disorder, which represents the form or the manner in which the child presents his or her thoughts to the listener. This includes:
  - illogical thinking
  - incoherence

- loose associations (when one thought does not logically relate to the next one)
- circumstantiality (delay in getting to the point because of unnecessary details)
- tangentiality (digressive, or irrelevant replies to questions, the responses never approaching the point of the questions)
- vague speech
- poverty of speech (short, limited and empty answers to questions)
- poverty of content (not having much to say about anything)
- echolalia (the immediate repeating of the words or sentence by the patient in response to a question just asked, parrot-like repetition)
- neologisms (making up new words)
- overelaborate speech
- thought blocking (halting speech in the middle of a sentence)

The DSM-IV-TR (2000) uses the term *disorganized speech* rather than formal thought disorder. Although any of these can be seen in normal people occasionally, it is the consistent and repeated presentation of these symptoms that characterizes a thought disorder.

- Hallucinations are defined as "false sensory perceptions not associated with real external stimuli" and as "an apparent perception of an external object when no object is present." Hallucinations may involve any of the five senses. Hallucinations may be visual, auditory, gustatory, olfactory or tactile with auditory ones being the most common. What they all have in common is that what is perceived is not occurring in reality. Hallucinations that occur in mental illnesses are different from those that appear when falling asleep (hypnagogic hallucinations) or while waking up (hypnopompic hallucinations). These are seen in normal people. In schizophrenia, hallucinations occur when the person is fully awake.

- Delusions are beliefs that appear as bizarre or false to other persons from the same culture. They cannot be changed by logic or clear evidence. Delusions can be difficult to assess but they seem to be present in at least 50% of the cases of schizophrenia. They are different from hallucinations in that the stimulus may exist in reality but the belief or interpretation that the patient makes is bizarre. For example, a child in school speaks to the teacher and the patient thinks that the child is reporting to the teacher something about him or that there is a conspiracy against him.

Hallucinations and delusions are sometimes called *content thought disorders*. Schizophrenia is a disease that presents with a psychotic thought process as described above but also with abnormal behaviors (disorganized, bizarre, inappropriate or catatonic posturing, rigidity, excitement), negative symptoms, social dysfunction and of a duration of at least six months.

3. Is my child insane?

First let's define the word *insane*. It is actually a very old word in English and the dictionary definition in the *Merriam-Webster Dictionary* is "a deranged state of mind usually occurring as a specific disorder." It is now primarily a legal term used in court to indicate being unable to control or understand the illegality of one's actions. *Insane* is not a term used in regular speech.

Many changes have been made in the way childhood schizophrenia has been described and diagnosed. At first, only adults were considered to have schizophrenia.

Many changes have been made in the way childhood schizophrenia has been described and diagnosed.

The Basics

Psychiatrist

A medical doctor, specializing in the diagnosis and treatment of mental illnesses and emotional problems.

Insanity

Mental malfunctioning or unsoundness of mind to produce lack of judgment and to the degree that the individual cannot determine right from wrong.

In the mid-19th century, Maudsley (a famous British **psychiatrist**) was discussing **insanity**. By the late 19th century, Kraeplin used the term *dementia praecox* to describe a severe disorder that sometimes started in childhood. Kraeplin and Bleuler thought that schizophrenia presented in a similar form during childhood and adolescence, though more rarely. De Sanctis (1906) proposed the term *dementia praecoccissima*. Because the diagnosis in children was less common than in adults and more difficult to characterize, it was called *childhood psychosis* and childhood schizophrenia was a diagnosis that included all psychotic children.

There was a major controversy over the relationship of childhood psychosis to adult schizophrenia dating to the 1940s and Kanner's description of early infantile autism. Because autism is a severe psychiatric disorder with a very early onset, it was thought to be the earliest manifestation of adult schizophrenia. It was only in the 1970s that the differentiation was made between infantile autism and childhood schizophrenia and it was understood that the disorders can be unrelated. Some authors call for a broader definition of the concept of childhood schizophrenia with the creation of a larger spectrum of these disorders.

There are subgroups of children within the schizophrenia spectrum who do not meet the full criteria for a complete diagnosis of childhood schizophrenia, but who do present with complex developmental disorders and possible psychotic symptoms. Some other labels have been proposed:

Bipolar

A psychiatric condition characterized by mood swings that occur episodically.

- Multi-dimensionally impaired (MDI). These children have neither **bipolar** disorder nor schizophrenia, but experience short psychotic episodes, attention problems, and unstable moods.

- **Pervasive developmental disorders** not otherwise specified (PDD-NOS). PDD-NOS is used when a child has symptoms of autism but not in the configuration needed for an autism diagnosis. The social component is where the most impairment is seen.
- Multiplex developmental disorders (MDD). Children who display the severe, early-appearing social and communicative deficits characteristic of autism, but who also display some of the emotional instability and disordered thought processes that resemble schizophrenic symptoms.

More research is needed to understand and differentiate these disorders.

It should be noted that it is only since 1980 that the more narrow and conservative view of childhood schizophrenia under DSM-IV has been in use.

The conventional definition is that early-onset schizophrenia (EOS) has its onset before age 18 years, and very-early-onset schizophrenia (VEOS) develops before age 13 years.

Pervasive developmental disorders

Refers to a group of five disorders characterized by delays in the development of multiple basic functions including socialization and communication.

The Basics

PART TWO

Signs & Symptoms: The Diagnosis

My child is absolutely convinced that someone is following him. What does this mean?

Earlier, you described the positive symptoms like hallucinations. But what are the negative symptoms?

What is the frequency of childhood schizophrenia?

More . . .

4. My child says that he hears voices. What does this mean?

Hallucinations may be more or less vivid and, by themselves, hallucinations do not define schizophrenia or psychosis. They can be found in normal children suffering from anxiety, responding to acute stress or deprivation and mood disorders (depression, bipolar disorders).

Presuming there are no voices, your child is having a hallucination. Hallucinations may be more or less vivid and, by themselves, hallucinations do not define schizophrenia or psychosis. They can be found in normal children suffering from anxiety, responding to acute stress or deprivation and mood disorders (**depression**, bipolar disorders).

In childhood schizophrenia, about 80% of cases report auditory hallucinations, making it the most frequently reported symptom.

They may include persecutory or **command hallucinations**, conversing voices or voices making comments about the child. Visual and somatic hallucinations (olfactory, tactile, gustatory hallucinations) are less frequent.

Hallucinations appear to be rare in children younger than 6 or 7 years of age. Auditory hallucinations reported by children can be:

"The voices are telling me to kill myself."

"The voices are telling me to run away."

"The voices are telling me to do bad things."

"The voices are telling me to kill someone."

"The voices are telling me to steal."

"The voices are telling me to break things."

"Voices are calling me bad names."

"A voice is telling me to do good things."

"A voice is calling my name."

Depression

A major psychiatric condition characterized by profound sadness all day.

Command hallucinations

Imaginary voices that tell the hearer what to do.

"I hear the voices of two people arguing."

"I hear the voice of a monster."

"I hear a mumbling voice."

The voices may be talking about the child in a derogatory manner. They can talk to each other or comment on the child's actions. In the majority of cases the voices are negative.

Sometimes, the voice is from somebody that the child knows, but sometimes, it cannot be recognized. The voice may be from someone who is dead. Auditory hallucinations can be perceived as coming from inside the child's head or from outside. The voices may sound as real as an actual voice. Sometimes they come from no apparent source, other times they come from real people who aren't actually saying anything. Children may have difficulties accurately describing the location of the hallucinations. Sometimes, the child may be found talking to himself.

Visual hallucinations are less frequent (30% to 79%) and are usually about people, monsters, fantasy figures, animals, shadows, shapes, scenes or scary figures.

Much more rare are olfactory hallucinations (21%) or tactile (37%). These are frequently due to substance abuse or an organic neurological problem and thus may not be part of schizophrenia.

Command hallucinations (where the voice orders the child to do something) can be very disturbing and lead to dangerous behaviors such as **suicide** or **homicide**. Their presence may oblige the physician to hospitalize the child on an emergency basis.

Suicide

The act of causing ones own death.

Homicide

The killing of one human being by another human being.

15

From a mother:

*Renee, our 16-year-old daughter was found with her clothing torn up and exhausted, after walking 20 miles away from our house. The police found her and called me because we filed a missing person report 2 days ago. We rushed to the hospital where they took her. The psychiatrist in the emergency room told us that Renee said that she had been hearing male voices coming out of the telegraphic poles and lines, telling her to go to the city which is 200 miles away. That didn't make any sense. The voices were so loud that she felt that she didn't have a choice. They were telling her that she was on a mission and had to find the savior "so the little children of the world would be happy." We thought maybe she had been kidnapped and maybe even sexually abused but there were no marks on her and the doctors who examined her said she had not been abused. She also said no one touched her because she was the savior. We spoke with our minister to see if maybe this really was a religious vision but he did not think so. They started treating her with an **antipsychotic** medication and she's better. She says the voice has disappeared but I think she still believes she is the savior. I hope the medicine makes that go away soon.*

Antipsychotic

Any medication that specifically suppresses the positive symptoms of hallucinations and delusions.

Normal children, from the toddler years through adolescence, present their thoughts in a logical and coherent manner to the listener.

5. How is a thought disorder detected in a child?

Normal children, from the toddler years through adolescence, present their thoughts in a logical and coherent manner to the listener. Thought disorders have been described in 40% to 100% of children with schizophrenia. Magical thinking (the belief that thinking equals doing and that just thinking something causes it to happen) or illogical thinking, incoherence and loosening of associations are frequently observed. These are not specific to childhood-onset schizophrenia and can be seen in other illnesses, such as major depressions. In the early phase of the illness, the thought disorder may not meet the strict diagnostic criteria but as the child develops the remaining criteria are met. The assessment might also be problematic in very young children as well as in the developmentally delayed children. Tests have been developed to assess younger children. These include:

- The Interview for Childhood Disorders and Schizophrenia may be used. It was developed by Russell et al. (1989), who helped to demonstrate that in a sample of young schizophrenics, 40% showed incoherence, loosening of associations, illogical thinking and poverty of content.
- The Thought Disorder Index (TDI) was developed by Arboleda and Holzman (1985). They found that children with psychotic spectrum disorders and those at risk for schizophrenia had more severe thought disorder levels than normal children and children with nonpsychotic psychiatric diagnoses. Using the TDI, a study comparing schizophrenic adolescents to adolescents with psychotic depression and to adolescents with no mental illness found that a thought disorder was evident in both the adolescents with schizophrenia and those with psychosis. However, the content was more bizarre in the schizophrenic adolescents.
- A play procedure (the Story Game) and a coding system (the Kiddie Formal Thought Disorder Scale or KFTDS) was developed by Caplan for the assessment of formal thought disorders in middle childhood. Comparing schizophrenic, schizotypal (children with need for social isolation, odd behavior and thinking, and often unconventional beliefs) and normal children showed that loose associations occur almost exclusively in the schizophrenic and

the schizotypal children and not in the normal children. It is also to be noted that Caplan et al. (2000) found that normal children younger than 7 years of age may have illogical thinking and loose associations.
- Rorschach cards are also frequently used to elicit speech samples from children.

6. My child is absolutely convinced that someone is following him. What does this mean?

A delusion is a belief held with total conviction, one that has great personal significance to the individual and is not amenable to reason or modifiable by experience. Few studies have focused on delusions of children.

Paranoid and persecutory delusions are the most frequent. Children may think that:

Paranoid

Excessive or irrational suspicion or distrust of others.

- They are going to be poisoned with food.
- Someone is going to kill them.
- Someone is following them.
- Their bedroom has a camera and someone is watching them.
- People are talking about them, or looking at them.
- They are spied on (with tracking devices, implants).
- People are working together to harass them.
- Something is controlling them (for example with an electronic implant).
- People can read their mind or control their thoughts.
- Their thoughts are being broadcast over the radio or TV.
- Delusions that someone, often a famous person, is in love with the adolescent.

Other kinds of delusions exist:

- Somatic delusions might be present. The child may think that there is a baby in the belly or that someone has put a camera in the stomach.
- Delusions of reference. The child may think that random events have a special meaning. (e.g., that what is written in a book is a sign trying to tell the child something).
- Religious delusions. The child may think that they are the Messiah or a prophet.
- Delusions of grandeur. The child may believe that he or she has an important mission or is an unrecognized genius.

Delusions reported in childhood schizophrenia are similar to the ones in adult schizophrenia. Like adults, children may have delusions of control, sin, thought insertion (that people put thoughts in their mind), ideas of reference (people on TV shows are speaking about them), grandiose delusions, somatic delusions or bizarre delusions.

Unlike adults, a child's delusions may be less elaborate and take the form of irrational fears. Children may have magical thinking and morbid fantasies that can be fixated and pervasive. The child may have poor reality testing and not see the imaginary quality of these thoughts. These thoughts may be the precursors of delusions that will develop later.

The **incidence** of delusions in childhood schizophrenia reported in studies varies from 36% to 94%.

Delusions may also occur in children with major depressive disorders like depression and bipolar disorders.

Signs & Symptoms: The Diagnosis

Unlike adults, a child's delusions may be less elaborate and take the form of irrational fears.

Incidence

The term *incidence* of a disease refers to the annual diagnosis rate, or the number of new cases of that disease diagnosed each year.

This shows that delusions are not specific to child-hood schizophrenia.

In young children, or in those with developmental delays, severely abnormal thinking (delusions) may not be present, especially in the early phase of the illness. Even if symptoms are present, the limitations of normal cognitive development make it very difficult to identify psychotic symptoms reliably in children younger than seven.

From a father:

Marissa, our 17-year-old, thought that she had been raped and that she was pregnant. She also was saying that a camera was in her vagina and had recorded the event. She was very fearful that the recorded movie was going to be broadcast on television and put on the internet like on YouTube or Facebook. She was demanding to have a gynecologist remove the camera. We brought her to her gynecologist who examined her and confirmed, of course, that there was no camera. She also confirmed that Marissa was still a virgin and that she certainly was not pregnant. We are very scared about all of this and will be seeing a psychiatrist at the university medical center next week.

7. What are the different types of schizophrenia?

Different subtypes of schizophrenia have been described. One person may be diagnosed with different subtypes over the course of his or her illness. The symptoms may change within the same child as the disease progresses.

Paranoid Subtype

The defining feature is the presence of auditory hal-lucinations or delusional thoughts about persecution or conspiracy. People with this subtype may be more functional in their ability to work and engage in relationships than people with other subtypes of schizophrenia. The paranoid subtype usually appears later in life and patients have achieved a higher level of functioning before the onset of their illness. They may not appear odd or unusual. Typically, the hallucinations and delusions revolve around a theme that often remains consistent over time. Paranoid schizophrenics will often come to the attention of mental health professionals only when there has been some major stress in their life that has caused an increase in their symptoms. Since there may be no features observable to outsiders, the evaluation requires sufferers to be somewhat open to discussing their thoughts. If there is a significant degree of suspiciousness or paranoia present, the patient may be very reluctant to discuss these issues with a stranger, even a physician.

People with this subtype may be more functional in their ability to work and engage in relationships than people with other subtypes of schizophrenia.

There is a broad spectrum to the nature and severity of symptoms that may be present at any one time. When symptoms are in a phase of exacerbation, or worsening, there may be some disorganization of the thought processes (thoughts becoming illogical, vague).

From a father:

Jamal, at age 15, started to retreat into his room and stopped talking to us. He wouldn't eat dinner with the family—which I insist upon because this is quality time when my wife, the 3 kids, and I can all be together. Jamal was taking kitchen knives in his room and putting them under his bed. He said he was afraid his sister would kill him. He said that he knew it by the way she was looking at him and that this special look meant that she had a plan to kill him. Fortunately, my wife found the knives when she cleaned the room. Jamal told her why the knives were there and she called the police to bring him to the hospital. The examining psychiatrist said he was paranoid and they admitted him to the hospital for tests and treatment.

Disorganized Subtype

The predominant feature of the disorganized subtype is disorganization of the thought processes. Hallucinations and delusions may be less pronounced. These patients think differently from normal people and this abnormality may be reflected in other parts of their life. They may have significant impairments in their ability to maintain the activities of daily living. Even the more routine tasks, such as dressing, bathing, or brushing teeth, can be significantly impaired.

There is often impairment in the emotional processes of the individual. These patients may appear emotionally unstable or their emotions may not seem appropriate to the context of the situation. They may fail to show ordinary emotional responses in situations that evoke responses in healthy people. They have a blunted (showing no emotion) or an inappropriate affect (the emotion shown does not fit with what is discussed). For example, they laugh when talking about sad subjects or show indifference when talking about very personal issues.

Patients may also have significant impairment in their ability to communicate effectively. At times, their speech can become virtually incomprehensible, due to disorganized thinking. In the past, the term *hebephrenic* has been used to describe this subtype.

Catatonic Subtype

The predominant clinical features of the catatonic subtype involve disturbances in movement. Voluntary movement may stop, as in catatonic stupor. Alternatively, activity can dramatically increase, as in catatonic excitement. Purposeless actions repetitively performed (stereotypic behavior), may occur, with no productive activity. This may include waving of the arms, making noises or strange sounds, pacing up and down or other unusual actions. Thus the catatonic subtype does not always imply **catatonia** or total immobility. These disturbances may last from minutes to hours.

Patients may exhibit a resistance to any attempt to change how they appear. They may maintain a pose or position without moving, sometimes for long periods of time (waxy flexibility). They may voluntarily assume unusual body positions, or manifest unusual facial contortions or limb movements. Other symptoms include repeating what another person is saying (echolalia) or mimicking the movements of another person (echopraxia).

Catatonia

A condition that is characterized by extremes in behavior, of which the individual appears to be unaware.

Undifferentiated Subtype

In this subtype, people have symptoms that are not sufficiently formed or specific enough to permit classification of the illness into one of the other subtypes.

The symptoms of a patient can fluctuate at different points in time, resulting in uncertainty as to the correct subtype classification. Other people will exhibit symptoms that are remarkably stable over time but still may not fit one of the typical subtype pictures

In this subtype, people have symptoms that are not sufficiently formed or specific enough to permit classification of the illness into one of the other subtypes.

Residual Subtype

This subtype is diagnosed when the patient no longer displays severe symptoms. Hallucinations, delusions or idiosyncratic behaviors may still be present, but significantly diminished in comparison to the acute phase of the illness. These patients often have little interest in life and do not do well with interactions with other people. They may avoid eye contact or conversation with others.

Although all subtypes can occur in adolescence, there is a predominance of the disorganized and undifferentiated subtypes.

8. Is my child less intelligent because of schizophrenia?

Children with schizophrenia usually perform in the low average to normal range of intelligence. However, there are reports of a significant decline in full-scale Intelligence Quotient (IQ) scores in children with schizophrenia when measured prior to and following the onset of psychosis. This is probably either due to the inability to make age-appropriate developmental gains or due to the ongoing pathological process. It was also reported that people who start with a higher IQ may decompensate less when they have a psychotic episode.

When comparing a group of children with childhood schizophrenia and high-functioning autistic children the full scale IQs did not differ. However, the schizophrenic children seemed to be more distractible than the autistic children.

Several studies of children have found a mean IQ of between 80 and 85 (which is below the general population mean), with about one-third of cases having an IQ lower than 70. This represents a mean IQ score about 10 points lower than those reported in studies of adult schizophrenia.

There are, unfortunately, many unanswered questions. Those questions are:

- Which deficits precede the onset of psychosis?
- Are the deficits a consequence of the psychosis?
- Is the pattern of deficits specific to schizophrenia or shared with other developmental disorders?
- Are the cognitive impairments progressive or static?

Adolescents with schizophrenia have particular difficulties with short-term **working memory**, selective and sustained attention, and speed of processing information. A good understanding of the specific cognitive deficits in an individual can be very helpful in guiding education and rehabilitation. Tasks will need to be broken down into small more manageable parts.

Working memory
This is a more contemporary term for short-term memory.

9. My adolescent stays in his room all the time and does not communicate with us. Is this normal in that age group? Is he lazy? Is he depressed?

In adolescence, although moods frequently fluctuate, children are still involved with their family and friends. They still continue normal activities like school and hobbies and they enjoy life and friends. A dramatic change in a child's behavior and functioning, however, is an alarm signal. Generally, schizophrenia develops progressively over a period of 6 months to 2 years. Family and friends notice some changes in the child's behavior, such as becoming inattentive, irritable, and withdrawing from them. The adolescent may sleep too much or too little. He may get agitated for no apparent reason. Sometimes, the adolescent makes strange statements that are not true about people or events that he thinks have actually happened. He may be

In adolescence, although moods frequently fluctuate, children are still involved with their family and friends. They still continue normal activities like school and hobbies and they enjoy life and friends. A dramatic change in a child's behavior and functioning, however, is an alarm signal.

heard talking to himself. He may be involved in strange activities in his room, like praying, chanting, or researching strange subjects on the internet. Normal hygiene routines may not be followed. The adolescent may begin hoarding food or other objects in his room for some unknown reason. Refusing to go to school may become an issue.

It may appear that the child is depressed or oppositional, which may delay the correct diagnosis of schizophrenia. A consultation with the family doctor or pediatrician might not be enough if their opinion is that the child will grow out of it and that this is just adolescence. A consultation with a child psychiatrist may be needed, possibly with follow-up visit if the first evaluation does not give a definitive answer.

The adolescent who is developing schizophrenia usually has no insight about being ill and may not tell his family, friends, or his physician that he has disturbing, confusing thoughts or hallucinations. A trustful relationship with the doctor will be needed to reveal these internal preoccupations and to allow the possibility of treatment.

10. Earlier, you described the positive symptoms like hallucinations. But what are the negative symptoms?

The negative symptoms are less dramatic but more pernicious. They include:

- Affective flattening (lack or decline in emotional response)
- Alogia (lack or decline in speech)
- Avolition (lack or decline in motivation)

These can include a cluster called the 4 A's:

- Autism (loss of interest in other people or the surroundings)
- Ambivalence (emotional withdrawal)
- Blunted affect (a bland and unchanging facial expression)
- Loose association (cognitive problems in which people join thoughts without clear logic, frequently jumbling words together into a meaningless "word salad")

Other common symptoms include a lack of spontaneity, impoverished speech, difficulty establishing rapport, and a slowing of movement. Apathy and lack of interest can cause friction between children and their parents, who may view these attributes as signs of laziness rather than manifestations of the illness.

When children with schizophrenia are evaluated with pencil-and-paper psychological tests designed to detect brain injury, they show a pattern suggestive of widespread dysfunction. Virtually all aspects of brain operation from the simplest basic sensory processes to the most complex aspects of thought are affected to some extent. Certain functions, such as the ability to form new memories (either temporarily or permanently) or to solve complex problems may be particularly impaired. Patients may display difficulty solving ordinary problems encountered in daily living, and this may account for the difficulty such individuals have in living independently later on.

Overall, schizophrenia conspires to rob people of the very qualities they need to thrive in society: personality, social skills, and wit.

Apathy and lack of interest can cause friction between children and their parents, who may view these attributes as signs of laziness rather than manifestations of the illness.

Signs & Symptoms: The Diagnosis

11. My child has admitted to using illicit drugs. Can he become psychotic or even schizophrenic because of this?

Many drugs can cause psychotic-like symptoms.

• Cannabis (Hash, Marijuana)

Frequent cannabis use during adolescence and young adulthood raises the risk of psychotic symptoms later in life. The proportion of young people who have used cannabis has increased and the age of first use has declined. A study in Sweden found that people who had used cannabis more than 50 times before the age of 18 were three times more likely to develop schizophrenia.

The strength of cannabis being sold now is higher than the strength of the drug sold during the 1960s and 1970s. THC levels are thought to have doubled in the most popular type of street cannabis. Exposure to cannabis quadrupled in the 30 years prior to 2002 and it is used 18 times more frequently in children under eighteen. This increased exposure to more potent drugs may be quite harmful.

Dopamine

A chemical substance that is important for conveying "messages" between nerve cells in the brain.

The risk of developing schizophrenia is much higher in young people who are already genetically vulnerable to developing psychosis. Cannabis may disrupt the balance of the chemical **dopamine** in the brain. Because many people who use marijuana do not become schizophrenic, there is probably a genetic predisposition to developing the illness in some people. That is, the drug use may bring out a genetically predetermined illness in one of two ways. It can either lower the age symptoms first appear or bring the disease out in someone whose genetic predisposition is only mild to moderate and who might not have developed it without this added stimulus.

Cannabis use seems to be associated with the onset of schizophrenia at a younger age, a worse outcome, and is seen more frequently in males, who tend to use greater quantities than females do. **Risk factors** mentioned for developing a schizophrenia-spectrum illness from marijuana use include a family history of psychosis, frequent use, or having unusual or psychotic-like experiences from the marijuana. In a New Zealand study, young people with a variant allele of the COMT **gene** (a type of **DNA** sequence) who used cannabis had a risk of reporting psychotic symptoms that was ten times higher than young people who did not have the allele and used cannabis.

Although it is not known whether cannabis can actually cause true schizophrenia, it is clear that it can produce psychosis and schizophrenic-like symptoms. Some feel that cannabis and other drugs may push the child from schizophrenic-like symptoms into frank schizophrenia if there is a genetic predisposition.

From Carlos's dad:

Carlos was paranoid and could not go to sleep. His best help was to smoke some weed every night. It helped him to feel calmer, more relaxed. It is only when medications started working that he did not feel the need to use his daily joint.

- PCP (phencyclidine) or Angel Dust

   Phencyclidine (PCP), a hallucinogenic drug, has caused psychosis in normal research volunteers and exacerbates psychotic symptoms in patients with schizophrenia present already.

   PCP induces symptoms that resemble negative and cognitive symptoms of schizophrenia as well as positive ones. These effects are seen not just in abusers

Risk factors
A characteristic that increases a person's likelihood of developing a disorder.

Gene
A functional unit of heredity that is in a fixed place in the structure of a chromosome.

Although it is not known whether cannabis can actually cause true schizophrenia, it is clear that it can produce psychosis and schizophrenic-like symptoms.

DNA
DNA is made of different nucleic acids: adenine, guanine, thiamine, and cytosine and is put together in the form of a triple helical structure.

of PCP but also in individuals given brief, low doses of PCP or ketamine (an anesthetic with similar effects) in research trials. Individuals receiving PCP exhibited the same type of disturbances in performing interpretation tests as those with schizophrenia.

• Amphetamines (Speed or Ecstasy)

Amphetamines are known to induce hallucinations and delusions in habitual abusers. They stimulate dopamine release in the brain, which is linked to psychosis (see question 29 on the Dopamine Hypothesis). High doses of amphetamines may cause schizophrenic-like symptoms (amphetamine psychosis). In addition, amphetamines may worsen the symptoms of patients who already have schizophrenia.

• LSD (lysergic acid dietylamide)

LSD is a hallucinogen in normal individuals. It is clear that LSD is able to produce psychosis, though the debate is whether these people were predisposed to develop psychosis or whether this occurred in normal (nonpredisposed) individuals. Similarly, a schizophrenic-like syndrome may be seen after LSD use. Some studies have suggested that the mechanism of LSD-induced symptoms may be a key to understanding the symptoms seen in nondrug induced schizophrenia.

What comes first, the use of drugs or the first symptoms of schizophrenia?

Sometimes, the use of illicit drugs is blamed for the diagnosis of psychosis or schizophrenia when, in fact, a child with schizophrenia may be using drugs and the diagnosis of schizophrenia has been missed. That is, the schizophrenia has been present for some time but the symptoms were missed.

Some researchers have suggested that cannabis-induced psychosis and schizophrenia are one and the same disease and that these people would have developed schizophrenia whether or not they used cannabis. Anyone who experiences a psychotic episode that lasts more than 48 hours after using marijuana should get immediate help as it may represent an opportunity for early diagnosis and treatment of schizophrenia and, therefore, a better **prognosis**.

Prognosis
Prediction of how a patient will progress.

12. My child was diagnosed with schizophrenia and is using marijuana. What are the risks?

- Substance use disorder (SUD) plays a prominent role in the cause, and the course of mental illnesses.
- Marijuana worsens psychotic symptoms of schizophrenics.
- Poor compliance with medical treatment is frequent if there is associated marijuana use.
- Multidrug use is a risk. Regular users of cannabis are more likely to use heroin, cocaine, or other drugs because they are in social environments that provide more opportunities to use these drugs. The earlier the age of first cannabis use, the more likely a young person is to use other illicit drugs. It is also possible that regular cannabis use produces changes in brain function that make the use of other drugs more attractive.
- In some cases, cannabis may be used to self-medicate against the symptoms of schizophrenia. However, the self-medication hypothesis was not supported in some studies which found that early

psychotic symptoms did not predict an increased use of cannabis. Another study found that cannabis users were more likely to report unusual perceptions after using cannabis than to use cannabis in response to experiencing unusual perceptions from some other cause.

The conclusions from these studies are that cannabis use, as well as other illicit drug use, is not advisable in people who have schizophrenia or some other psychosis or in people who may be at risk to developing such diseases. Given that these drugs have bad effects on other organs in the body, it is probably wise to avoid them altogether.

It should also be noted that street drugs are often mixed with other substances and fillers, which may be quite toxic also.

It should also be noted that street drugs are often mixed with other substances and fillers, which may be quite toxic also.

13. What if my child who has schizophrenia goes to a party and drinks alcohol?

People with mental disorders who are also taking psychotropic medications should not drink alcohol. It may exacerbate the symptoms of schizophrenia and lead to noncompliance with the treatment. Knowing that alcohol and medications can have interactions may lead the adolescent to stop his medicine to be able to drink at a party. Alcohol may increase the sedative effect of the psychotropic medications.

Patients with schizophrenia have higher rates of alcohol abuse disorders and schizophrenics who also have alcohol abuse disorders have less favorable courses and outcomes. In one study subjects with schizophrenia reported greater euphoria and stimulatory effects with alcohol. Some patients report temporary increases in positive psychotic symptoms and perceptual alterations.

It is clear that in patients with schizophrenia, alcohol use should be avoided or kept to a minimum.

14. What are the risks of smoking?

While the **prevalence** of smoking in the total U.S. population is about 25% to 30%, the prevalence among people with schizophrenia is about three times higher at almost 90%.

The relationship between smoking and schizophrenia is complex. It appears that there are both positive and negative effects of nicotine on a person who has schizophrenia and on the course of schizophrenia. It may be that nicotine is used as a means by those with schizophrenia to improve difficulties with attention, **cognition**, and information processing as well as decreasing the **side effects** of antipsychotic medications (e.g., abnormal movements such as extra-pyramidal effects).

In schizophrenic patients, nicotine has been shown to help with some cognitive problems, to improve the person's ability to make sense of environmental stimuli and to improve concentration. Schizophrenic patients have changes in their nicotine **receptors** (expression, distribution, and function) in the brain. Research on nicotine receptors and possible nicotine use in schizophrenia treatment are currently being explored.

The major downside to smoking by schizophrenics is the same as that in the general population. Smoking is a direct cause of cancer and this might be a reason why

Prevalence

The term *prevalence* of a disease usually refers to the estimated population of people who are living with that disease at any given time.

Cognition

The quality of the mind that allows animals to think, reason, and manipulate their environment to survive.

Side effects

An unintended effect of a drug.

Receptors

A molecule that recognizes a specific chemical.

Signs & Symptoms: The Diagnosis

life expectancy for people with schizophrenia is about 20% shorter than for people who do not have schizophrenia. There is also high risk for diabetes, lung diseases, and other cancers in smokers. Smoking has also been found to interfere with the response to antipsychotic drugs. Schizophrenia patients who smoke need higher doses of antipsychotic medication. Finally, smoking is a large financial burden for people who have schizophrenia.

Schizophrenia patients who smoke need higher doses of antipsychotic medication.

15. What is the relationship between schizophrenia and epilepsy?

In a Danish study of more than two million people, those with epilepsy had about 2.5 times the risk of having schizophrenia as the general population.

A small percentage of epileptic patients experience psychotic symptoms during or after seizures, usually in the days or weeks after a seizure. Sometimes this resolves without developing into a chronic psychosis. This increased risk is not associated with any particular type of epilepsy.

Ictal

Physiologic state or event such as a seizure, stroke, or headache.

Remission

The state of absence of disease activity in patients with a chronic illness, with the possibility of return of disease activity.

Separate from the symptoms right at the time of the seizure, patients with epilepsy are also at increased risk for psychosis, which can be inter-**ictal** (in between epilepsy attacks), post-ictal (after a seizure), or , in rare cases, an expression of the seizure activity. This psychosis can be related to seizure **remission** (i.e., "alternative psychosis" or "forced normalization") or be due to the medical treatment (e.g., related to antiepileptic drugs or after brain surgery).

It can be difficult to distinguish between alternative psychosis and the psychosis that occasionally occurs as a side effect of most seizure medicines. Alternative psychosis is an unusual type of psychosis in people with epilepsy which occurs when seizures are well controlled by seizure medicines and their EEG becomes normal. The psychotic symptoms are inversely related to the occurrence of seizures, generally in people who have had epilepsy for a long time. Treatment of any of the psychoses of epilepsy should take this phenomenon into account. Treatment with antiseizure drugs may stop the seizures but worsen the behavior of the patients. The mechanism underlying these interesting phenomena is not yet understood.

The connection of psychosis to epilepsy is interesting because it may provide new insights into the causes of each disease and pathways for treatment. Prescribing antiepileptic/anticonvulsant medications is already common practice when treating "treatment resistant schizophrenia" (that is, patients resistant to the classic antipsychotic drug treatments). The antiepileptic medications have been shown in some people to decrease irritability, positive symptoms, anxiety, or aggressive behaviors.

In studying the relationship between epilepsy and psychiatric disorders, care must be taken to differentiate between the following:

- Psychiatric disorders caused by the seizures—Ictal disorders, post-ictal disorders, and inter-ictal disorders.
- Epileptic and psychiatric disorders caused by common brain pathology (such as brain tumors or toxins).
- Epileptic and psychiatric disorders that happen to coexist in the same patient but are not causally related (e.g., a schizophrenic patient who has an auto accident and develops epilepsy due to head trauma).

Antidepressants

A medication used to treat depression.

To be noted: **antidepressants** and antipsychotic drugs have the potential to increase seizures by lowering the seizure threshold (the point at which a patient has a seizure).

16. What is the frequency of childhood schizophrenia?

Due to changes in the diagnostic criteria over the years, studies have been very difficult to interpret. One problem in giving accurate information on the frequency of childhood schizophrenia is that many children receiving the diagnosis of schizophrenia do not meet the criteria for schizophrenia and may be misdiagnosed. A large proportion might have another diagnosis such as depression with psychotic features.

Schizophrenia appears to be less frequent than autism. A 1971 study found autism to be 1.4 times as common as childhood schizophrenia and affects about 1 in 500 children. Childhood schizophrenia affects only about 1 in 40,000 children compared to 1 in 100 adults.

Schizophrenia appears to be less frequent than autism. A 1971 study found autism to be 1.4 times as common as childhood schizophrenia and affects about 1 in 500 children. Childhood schizophrenia affects only about 1 in 40,000 children compared to 1 in 100 adults.

The prevalence of schizophrenia (the percentage of people with the disease in the general population at a particular point in time) is:

Monozygotic

Twins born at the same time who originate from the splitting of the same egg after it has been fertilized.

- In the general population: 1% (more than 3 million in the United States)
- In a nontwin brother or sister of a schizophrenia patient: 8%
- In a child with one parent with schizophrenia: 12%
- In a dizygotic twin (nonfraternal) of a schizophrenic patient: 12%
- In the child of two parents with schizophrenia: 40%
- In a **monozygotic** twin (fraternal) of a schizophrenic patient: 47%

17. What are the precursors, or early indications, of schizophrenia in childhood?

In some cases, there are early developmental differences in children who develop schizophrenia compared to those children who do not.

Schizophrenia, like autism, has roots in the development of the brain. The developmental damage is more common than in adult-onset schizophrenia. Research shows that 30% of these children show signs of developmental disorders in the first few years of life.

The early history of patients with childhood schizophrenia often includes significant deficits:

- Deficits in language: expression and comprehension.
- Reading difficulties.
- Deficits in motor functioning: poor coordination, delays in developmental milestones. These may be more frequent in boys than girls.
- Deficits in social functioning: social withdrawal, aloofness.
- Attention problems, hyperactivity.
- Problems in bladder control.

Frequently, children receive other psychiatric diagnoses before the diagnosis of schizophrenia is clearly made. Other diagnoses include depression, ADHD, **conduct disorders**, and Pervasive Development Disorders (PDD). Sometimes PDD may be diagnosed due to the presence of similar symptoms such as echolalia, aloofness, hand flapping.

Poor school performance is frequently associated with childhood schizophrenia, even prior to the onset of psychotic symptoms. Many children with schizophrenia

Conduct disorders
A disorder where there is a repetitive pattern of not conforming to rules and social norms.

Signs & Symptoms: The Diagnosis

repeated grades, were put in special education classes or were diagnosed with learning disabilities.

It seems also that language impairment is more frequent in childhood-onset schizophrenia while impairment in social or motor functioning is more frequent in adolescent-onset schizophrenia.

It is suggested that the children with pre-morbid social and developmental impairments may have similar neurobiological defects as those with negative symptoms and poor adult outcome.

18. What is the age of onset and how does it start?

Schizophrenia is a disease that typically begins in adolescence or early adulthood, between the ages of 15 and 25.

Schizophrenia is a disease that typically begins in adolescence or early adulthood, between the ages of 15 years and 25 years. Men tend to develop schizophrenia slightly earlier than women. Schizophrenia onset is quite rare in patients younger than 10 years or older than 40 years of age. Only about 2% of adults with schizophrenia had the onset of their disease in childhood.

Childhood schizophrenia is seen as an early onset version of the adult disease but which stems from a more severe brain disruption.

Childhood schizophrenia is rarely diagnosed before 5 years of age. The onset for autism is usually around 3 years of age. The incidence of the disease increases slowly between ages 5 and 10 years. Between the ages of 10 and 15 years, the incidence of the diagnosis increases more rapidly and then reaches the adult level after age 15 years.

In a 1994 study, the mean age of onset of emotional disturbance was 4.6 years, the mean age of onset of actual psychotic symptoms was 6.9 years and the diagnosis of the full schizophrenic disorder was 9.5 years. This suggests a gradual onset of early, nonpsychotic symptoms, such as behavioral problems or mood instability, which progress to frank psychosis and then a more clear diagnosis.

Three classic patterns of disease onset have been described as:

- Acute onset without any previous evidence of disease.
- Insidious onset with a gradual deterioration in functioning.
- Insidious onset with an acute exacerbation (worsening) of the symptoms.

The insidious pattern of onset is the most frequent. It frequently starts with developmental, behavioral and psychiatric problems, followed a few years later by the appearance of psychotic symptoms.

Psychiatrists tend to differentiate very early onset in childhood (VEOS) from early onset in adolescence (EOS). Very Early Onset Schizophrenia (VEOS) in young children generally has an insidious onset rather than an acute, sudden presentation. In contrast, in adolescents (EOS), both acute onset (disease development in less than 1 year) and insidious onset (slower, longer course disease development) are seen.

The earlier the onset, the more severe and difficult the course of the disease.

Whether in a child or an adolescent, a critical sign to recognize is a change in the child or adolescent's functioning. The child becomes isolated. Their behavior may become erratic. Vague or different

Whether in a child or an adolescent, a critical sign to recognize is a change in the child or adolescent's functioning.

speech may develop; there may be involvement in philosophy or religion that seems out of the ordinary; there may be worsening of academic results; bizarre statements about friends or teachers; impulsive acts, irritability, agitation, and changes in sleep patterns. These early negative symptoms frequently have their onset well before the positive symptoms develop.

19. Is schizophrenia different in boys and girls?

Boys seem to have an onset earlier in childhood as well as to show early signs of abnormal development. They may also have a more insidious onset than girls. In some studies girls who develop schizophrenia were reported to be more introverted from kindergarten into adolescence whereas boys did not appear so in early grades but later were described as "disagreeable," in grades 7 to 12.

20. What is the course of the illness?

When the disease is treated, many of the symptoms may disappear or lighten but there may be significant residual symptoms that never disappear.

Usually there is a prodromal phase of schizophrenia. This is defined as a period before the development of the actual disease. It may be characterized by mild or different symptoms. It develops gradually, sometimes over a 2-year period. Then, there is an active phase of the disease with psychotic symptoms. When the disease is treated, many of the symptoms may disappear or lighten but there may be significant residual symptoms that never disappear.

In a study with more than 20 years of follow-up, 20% of the cases apparently had a complete remission. About 30% improved and the remaining 50% had moderate to poor outcomes, including some suicides.

Early onset (before the age of 10 years) in children with pre-morbid personality difficulties (behavioral and emotional problems prior to the evidence of psychosis) was of the worst prognosis.

Wide variation occurs in the clinical course of schizophrenia. Many children diagnosed with schizophrenia show chronic difficulties, such as:

- Fewer close social relationships
- Less academic achievement
- More unemployment
- Less capacity for independent living

Without treatment, the natural course of schizophrenia is deterioration and chronic disabling symptoms. Early-onset schizophrenia can be understood as a progressive-deteriorating developmental disorder.

One of the issues that has become more difficult is the ability to predict the course of the disease. The ability to diagnose the disease has improved and there are now more effective, proactive treatments, so the course of the illness may have changed compared to what was seen 30 or 40 years ago.

If medications are stopped, the risk of relapse is extremely high.

Many patients do well, with minimal or no symptoms, if they are treated very early and consistently with medications. They will need strong support systems, continued treatment and close follow-up over their lifespan. If medications are stopped, the risk of **relapse** is extremely high.

Relapse

Occurs when a person is affected again by a condition that affected them in the past.

The time until relapse is variable but the relapse may be more difficult to treat and residual symptoms may be worse than after the initial episode. If medication for schizophrenia is discontinued, the relapse rate is about 80% within 2 years. With continued drug treatment, only about 40% of recovered patients will suffer relapses. Thus, it is critical to continue the medications unless the treating psychiatrist has good reason to discontinue therapy.

Schizophrenia is lifetime disorder but it can be treated.

It is very important to educate patients and families so that patients do not stop their treatments. If they do, getting the symptoms under control again may require hospitalization. Some patients have multiple, recurrent short-term hospitalizations, sometimes called revolving-door phenomena, or even long-term hospitalizations. Schizophrenia is a lifetime disorder but it can be treated.

Early intervention and early use of new medications lead to better medical outcomes. Recent research shows that the disease process of schizophrenia gradually and significantly damages the brain and that earlier treatments may result in less brain damage over time. The earlier someone with schizophrenia is diagnosed and stabilized on treatment, the better the long-term prognosis is for their illness. In adolescents, if a full recovery occurs, it is most likely to happen in the first 3 months of the illness. After 6 months of psychosis, the prognosis for a full recovery is poor. The best predictor of remission is what happens in the first 6 months.

Teen suicide is a growing problem—and teens with schizophrenia have approximately a 50% risk of attempted suicide.

The predictors of poor outcome in adolescent psychoses are:

- Poor functioning prior to the appearance of the psychosis
- Negative symptoms
- Disorganization of the thought process
- The duration of the untreated psychosis (DUP)

The predictors of a good outcome in adolescent psychoses are:

- Disappearance of symptoms within 3 to 6 months of onset
- Good functioning (at school, with friends) prior to the psychotic break

21. Are there laboratory tests, X-rays, scans, or biological markers of schizophrenia?

Unfortunately, there is no specific test or biological marker. Studies have shown that there are frequent signs of neurological immaturity such as delays in motor development and soft neurological signs, such as:

Unfortunately, there is no specific test or biological marker.

- Integrative sensory function: impaired audio and visual integration, impaired ability to discriminate between sharp and dull objects touching the skin (graphesthesia) and inability to identify objects by touch if not seeing them (astereognosis).
- Motor coordination: intention tremor (a tremor seen only on movement or doing something but not at rest), abnormalities in finger-thumb opposition and coordination, in balance and gait.
- Motor sequencing: poor performance in complex motor tasks like repetitive alternating hand positions.

Some children with schizophrenia have hypotonia (low muscle tone) and hyporeflexia (below normal or absent reflexes). Sometimes, abnormalities in the EEG (brain waves) or autonomic nervous system activity (abnormalities in skin conductance and heart rate) are seen.

Some areas of studies have shown interesting results and may ultimately lead to objective laboratory tests for schizophrenia.

- Smooth pursuit eye movements (eye tracking studies). Eye tracking is the ability of the eyes to follow moving objects. Abnormal eye-tracking is the inability for the eyes to follow moving targets *smoothly*. People with abnormal eye-tracking follow objects using saccadic or jerky eye movements. This condition is found in more than 50% of schizophrenics, as compared to only 8% of the general population. Abnormalities in eye movements and the inability to concentrate one's attention over sustained periods have been linked with schizophrenia.

Electroencephalo-gram

A type of test whereby electrodes are placed on several areas of the head and recordings are made of the brain's electrical activity.

- EEG Measurement of Sensory Processing. Many stimuli, such as auditory or visual, presented to an individual will elicit an evoked response, or event related potential, on the EEG (**electroencephalogram** which register the electrical waves of the brain). In schizophrenia, there is a sensory-processing deficit, which can be studied on the EEG by looking at evoked responses. For example, a positive waveform recorded in the EEG approximately 50 milliseconds after an auditory click stimulus is called the P50. In schizophrenic patients, abnormal P50 have been seen.

Elevated P50 ratios and anticipatory saccades may represent markers of the genetic risk for childhood schizophrenia.

Brain structure and anatomy. Children with schizophrenia have been studied with **MRI** (magnetic resonance imaging) scans and were found to have:

- Smaller total cerebral (brain) volume.
- Increased ventricular (fluid filled areas of the brain) volume.
- Smaller areas in the **thalamus** (a part of the brain responsible for processing sensory inputs, such as hearing, smelling, seeing, to get them ready for delivery to the upper part of the brain where their meanings are understood).
- Some changes in temporal lobe structures (parts of the brain where memory, speech and hearing inputs are handled).
- A progressive increase in ventricular size was seen in these subjects over a 2-year period.
- In comparison to normal controls, youths with VEOS had a four-times greater decrease in cortical gray brain matter volume during adolescence.

It is possible that these and other laboratory tests will lead to the development of one or more tests to make the diagnosis and follow the effectiveness of treatments. However, this is still a long way off.

Perhaps the most important finding to come out of recent research is that no one area of the brain is fully responsible for schizophrenia. Just as normal behavior requires the concerted action of the entire brain, the disruption of function in schizophrenia must be seen as a breakdown in functions both within and between different brain regions.

MRI

A method to examine the tissue of the brain using a magnetic field and computer system.

Thalamus

A brain structure that relays incoming sensory information.

Perhaps the most important finding to come out of recent research is that no one area of the brain is fully responsible for schizophrenia.

Signs & Symptoms: The Diagnosis

PART THREE

Causes of Schizophrenia

Are there any neuropsychological tests
for schizophrenia?

We have one child with schizophrenia. Should
we go and see a genetic counselor?

What laboratory tests are done and what
could they show?

More . . .

22. Can schizophrenia be caused by a virus?

The idea of a virus causing schizophrenia has been under consideration for a very long time. The evidence in favor of this hypothesis is that children born to mothers exposed to viruses during the second trimester of pregnancy, but not the first or third, have an increased risk for the development of schizophrenia.

There was an increase of schizophrenia admissions to hospitals after the influenza epidemic of 1918. Many viral infections have been considered, such as Cytomegalic, Herpes I and II, Epstein-Barr, and some Human Retroviruses.

No virus has been consistently isolated from the brain of schizophrenic people after death.

Against the hypothesis is the fact that in the majority of cases of schizophrenia there is no evidence of a viral cause or preceding infection. No virus has been consistently isolated from the brain of schizophrenic people after death.

It may be that the virus in the mother causes physiological stress, which in turn leads to development of the disease. It is possible that a viral infection during the second trimester of the pregnancy, when the brain is in its key development period, makes the fetus more vulnerable to the development of schizophrenia later on. This hypothesis continues to be actively explored.

It is not clear whether viruses might be a cause of schizophrenia.

23. Are there any neuropsychological tests for schizophrenia?

All the studies have shown deficits in attention and in the processing of information. The children with schizophrenia perform more slowly on tasks that demand attention and on tasks that impact short-term memory and mental flexibility. They also show deficits in spatial organization. They may be less efficient in dealing with complex information. They seem to be more distractible.

In one study of seven variables, schizophrenic patients scored poorly on seven out of seven tests compared to depressed patients who scored poorly on only two out of seven. In another study, schizophrenic patients did more poorly on tests of attention, executive function (e.g., problem-solving, thinking flexibility, fluency, planning, and deductive reasoning), verbal memory, visual memory, motor skills, and visual-spatial perception. Their scores were worse than those patients having depression with psychosis and those patients having depression without psychotic process.

These tests are sometimes useful for assessing function and tracking severity over time (especially after treatment has begun) but are not useful in making the diagnosis of schizophrenia.

24. Is schizophrenia in children due to psychological trauma, problems in the family, or bad parenting?

There is no evidence that childhood schizophrenia is due to psychological trauma.

Many neuropsychiatric problems exist in these children very early on, even before the diagnosis of schizophrenia is made. These problems include neuro-sensory and neuro-motor deficits, disturbances in attention, impaired ability to organize or to process thoughts and difficulties in communicating ideas. It is frequently seen in retrospect that these children have experienced psychotic symptoms for years before it becomes evident to families or teachers. It is even possible that young children have psychotic symptoms but do not perceive or experience their symptoms as abnormal. It may only be later on, when there is a crisis in the child's life, that there is worsening of the previously described symptoms and that the diagnosis is made.

There is no evidence that "bad" parenting (or any sort of parenting) causes schizophrenia.

There is no evidence that "bad" parenting (or any sort of parenting) causes schizophrenia. Schizophrenia is a disease with multiple causes and significant genetic and developmental components. Nonetheless, parenting can play a role in the course of the disease. How the parents and family act and react can worsen or improve the course of the disease and the effectiveness of the medical treatments.

Some abnormal family dynamics have been described, particularly in adult studies. These studies described disturbances in communication such as giving double messages and high levels of expressed emotion (yelling, shouting, fighting, or critical or hostile comments). It is not clear if these unusual patterns of interactions cause schizophrenia, or if they are a result of the patient's disease.

The causes of child onset schizophrenia (COS) are external to the parents and caregivers. When a child has COS, the whole family is affected. Parents become confused and bewildered. This confusion sometimes comes across as frustration and anger. Children sometimes have episodes in which they are extremely angry with their parents. If parents overreact, the child may become hostile. Younger kids, who have a hard time articulating their needs, may appear naughty, oppositional, needy, or anxious. They may have long and frequent temper tantrums and parenting is not always easy.

Parents may be blamed by other family members for being too lenient toward the child or being too strict and not understanding. The mother and father may have a different understanding of the situation and of the attitude to take. This often produces tension in the couple. The clever child may also respond by playing one parent against the other for his or her own advantage.

Having a child with a chronic illness is difficult to handle and you will need all the support you can get—both familial and professional—to achieve positive results. The parents need to be united in order to be firm, supportive, and consistent in the rules for the child and in deciding upon the treatment course for their child.

To be clear though, the parents are not to blame for the disease any more than the child is to blame. Rather, good parenting and support will make everyone's life easier and help the child in the fight against schizophrenia.

25. What about the environment? Are there any toxins that may have caused schizophrenia in my child?

When physicians and toxicologists speak about environmental factors, they usually consider "everything other than genes."

Complications or exposure to toxins during pregnancy or labor and delivery have been examined as possible risk factors in adult schizophrenia studies but there is little work in childhood schizophrenia (**Table 2**).

Table 2   Obstetrical Factors

Pregnancy	Infections	Flu, Genital Herpes, Exposure to cats that have Toxoplasmosis Gondii (a parasite)	Antibodies produced by the mother in response to the infection cross the placenta and may react with the fetus's developing immune system.
	Toxins	Lead and Alcohol	Drinking alcohol while pregnant may alter the child's dopamine system and may increase the risk of developing schizophrenia.
			Lead may interfere with the growth of nerve cells in the baby's brain during a developmental period known as synaptogenesis, when brain cells make many connections to one another and may result in apoptosis (cell death).
		Use of painkillers (e.g., aspirin)	Unusually high risk of schizophrenia (11.1% and 8.9%, respectively) in a small group of children from mothers who were treated with morphine or opioid pain killers (was it due to the substance, or the medical condition of the mother, or unidentified factors).
		X-rays during pregnancy	Recent research has also shown that exposure of the brain to ionizing (X-ray) radiation early in childhood (before 5 years of age) is associated with an increased risk of schizophrenia later in life.
		Low folic acid	Low maternal folate and high maternal homocysteine levels may increase the risk for developing schizophrenia.
	Season of birth	Birth during winter and early spring	Low sunlight exposure and vitamin D deficiency has been postulated as a factor in causing schizophrenia.
	Stress	Body weight	Risk of obstetric complications or treatment of hypertension with diuretics during pregnancy, which can retard brain development has been postulated as a factor in schizophrenia.

Table 2   (*Continued*)

		Unwanted pregnancy	Unwanted pregnancy in a high risk of women with a history of psychosis was associated with adult schizophrenia-spectrum disorder in their offspring.
		Association between short-birth intervals between children and schizophrenia in the offspring	A possible role of the hypothalamic-pituitary-adrenal (HPA) axis which controls stress hormone levels, including cortisol, has been postulated.
		Social stresses	Upbringing, migration, social defeat, and discrimination.
	Older age of father		Higher levels of DNA damage in the sperm of older men.
Birth	Complications	Maternal-fetal Rhesus (Rh) blood incompatibility (i.e., mother and child have different blood Rh groups)	Possibly by increasing risk of hypoxia (oxygen shortage) to the developing fetal brain.
	Low birth weight		Nutritional factors in early life may contribute to the neuro-developmental deficit in schizophrenia.

Stressful life events may be a precipitating factor in children, as they might interact with biological predispositions for the disease. Whether they are an actual cause of the disease is less clear.

Children with schizophrenia are more likely to come from a low social economic status but it is not clear if this is due to the economic situation or some other specific factor found in such an environment (e.g., toxins) or in the social setting such as parents' mental illnesses and their poor functioning.

Stressful life events may be a precipitating factor in children, as they might interact with biological predispositions for the disease. Whether they are an actual cause of the disease is less clear.

The following diagram (**Figure 1**) displays the increased risk (or "odds ratio") that is associated with environmental factors that have been linked with schizophrenia. These numbers are developed by comparing the presence of each risk factor in patients with schizophrenia against other groups of individuals without schizophrenia. The higher the odds ratio number, the greater the presence of the risk factor in the schizophrenic group. Please know that this shows association but not causality. It is very hard to prove something causes an illness. It can be suggested that two things might be linked, and risk factors are only links. A risk factor is not a cause, it is only statistical data.

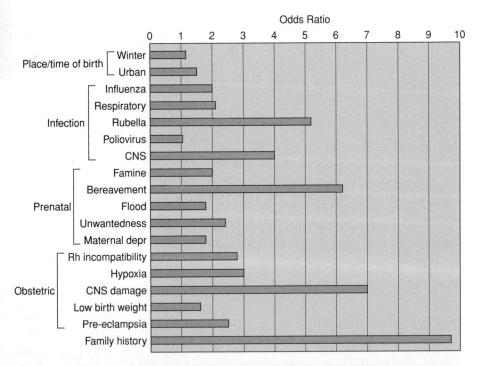

Figure 1 Comparison of a selected set of relatively well-established risk factors for schizophrenia, focusing mainly on pre- and antenatal factors [6]. (Abbreviations: CNS, central nervous system; depr, depression; Rh, Rhesus.) *Source:* Public Library of Science, Murray RM, Jones PB, Susser E, van Os J, Cannon M (2003) The epidemiology of schizophrenia. Cambridge: Cambridge University Press, p 470.

26. Is schizophrenia genetic? Is it inherited? What are the genetics involved?

There is some genetic predisposition to schizophrenia. Rates of schizophrenia among the first-degree relatives of children with schizophrenia are higher than normal. Rates of schizophrenia are elevated in relatives of adults with schizophrenia. Ten percent of the parents of children with schizophrenia have some kind of psychotic disorder. There may be an increased rate of mental retardation in the siblings of children with schizophrenia. In some cases, there was an association with abnormalities and we will talk about that later in this book.

There is some genetic predisposition to schizophrenia.

After a person has been diagnosed with schizophrenia, the chance of a sibling also being diagnosed with schizophrenia is 7% to 9%. If a parent has schizophrenia, the chance of a child having the disorder is 10% to 15%. Risks increase as the number of affected family members increases.

The correlation of schizophrenia between identical twins (who have identical genes) may be between 22.4% and 50%. This indicates that schizophrenia is *not* entirely a genetic disease but clearly has environmental components. In fact, it is felt that schizophrenia may not be a single disease with a single cause but is probably caused by a number of genetic and environmental factors interacting together.

Here is a brief summary of the genetics.

Human cells usually have 23 chromosome pairs. These are the long strands of DNA in cells that contain the genes. Each pair has one chromosome from the mother and one from the father. For pairs 1–22,

Causes of Schizophrenia

the chromosome is a copy of each parent's chromosome. In the final pair, there is an X chromosome from the mother, and either an X or Y chromosome from the father, for a total of 46.

A chromosome abnormality reflects a defect of chromosome number or structure. It occurs when there is an error in cell division and can be inherited from a parent or can occur on its own.

Deletions are shown when a portion of the chromosome is missing or deleted. Living organisms encode their genes in long strands of DNA.

Gene duplication is any duplication of a region of DNA that contains a gene. A gene is a portion of DNA which contains both coding sequences that determine what the gene does and noncoding sequences that determine when the gene is active or expressed.

Genetic studies developed tremendously with the Human Genome Project that ran from 1990–2003, focusing on the DNA sequence of an individual. A catalog of human genetic variation, called the HapMap was completed in 2005. To use the data, researchers compare large blocks of DNA sequence that tend to be inherited together (haplotypes) between people with and without a disease. Haplotypes shared by people with the disease are then examined in detail to look for associated genes.

There are many ways to look at chromosome studies:

Linkage

A genetic term that signifies a relationship between two or more genes on the same chromosome that are relatively close together so that sometimes the variations in the traits that each represents are inherited together in the same individual.

- Chromosomal **linkage** studies. Studies of two or more genes on the same chromosome that are close together and inherited together in the same individual. This helped to define genetic markers. These markers could be used to map the chromosomal location of different diseases.

- **Microarray** experiments. Chemical reaction that may also be used to test DNA fragments, antibodies, or proteins. These studies have been carried out in schizophrenia but it is still too early to conclude on the findings.
- Gene-association studies. These studies are done when researchers try to find out if a specific variation in a gene is more frequent in schizophrenic patients than in controls without the disease.

Many genes have been associated with schizophrenia by one of these methods:

Researchers from the Center for Human Genetic Research at Massachusetts General Hospital in Boston have found that deletions on chromosome 22q11.2, chromosomes 15q13.3, and 1q21.1 were associated with schizophrenia. Other researchers from Iceland have found similar deletions on chromosomes 15q13.3 and 1q21.1 as well as 15q11.2.

There is currently a lot of research on different genes.

- PRODH gene or proline dehydrogenase (located on 22q11.21)
- COMT gene or catechol-O-methyltransferase (located on 22q11.21-q11.23)
- DBH gene or dopamine beta-hydroxylase (located on 9q34)
- DDC gene or dopa decarboxylase (located on7p11)

Changes in these genes may affect the action of certain chemicals that transmit signals between **neurons** in

Microarray

This is an orderly arrangement of DNA samples to identify many genes at one time.

Causes of Schizophrenia

Neurons

A cell in the brain or nervous system that is specialized in sending, receiving, or processing information.

Neurotransmitters

A chemical which is a messenger within the brain.

the brain (**neurotransmitters**), resulting in an increased risk for psychiatric disorders

Multiple genes have been thought to be associated with schizophrenia (**Table 3**). It is possible that many of them may be necessarily present in one individual to be at risk for schizophrenia.

- Some genes may be acting on growth factors, brain growth and development, such as: BDNF (brain derived neurotrophic factor), AKT1 (proteine kinase).

Glutamate

An amino acid that is a building block of proteins.

- Some genes may be working on the **glutamate** pathway, like DTNBP1 (Dysbindin).
- Some others may be working on Dopaminergic and Serotonergic pathways, like COMT, DRD2, HTR2A.
- Some genes may be working on the circadian control, like CLOCK.
- Some may be working on cytokines (small proteins with a role in immune defense and neuromodulation in the CNS), like IL1B (Interleukins).
- Some may work on cortical development, like DISC1 (Disrupted in schizophrenia 1), PPP3CC (Calcineurin) or on **serotonin** receptors like YWHAH.

Serotonin

A hormone found in the brain, platelets, digestive tract, and pineal gland.

All of this is still very poorly understood and it is very likely that things will change as science furthers its knowledge.

Chromosome 22q11 deletion syndrome is associated with significantly increased risk for psychosis, predominantly schizophrenia. This syndrome is present in approximately 1 in 4000 births and a child born with it is 25 times more likely to have schizophrenia.

Table 3   Genes That Have Been Claimed Being Associated with Schizophrenia

Genes Functions	Genes Symbols
PI3K/AKT signaling growth factors, brain growth, and development	AKT1 (Protein kinase B), **BDNF** (brain derived neurotrophic factor) EGFR, GSK3B, IMPA2, NCAM1, **NRG1** (**Neuregulin -1**), PIK3C3, PIP5K2A, PDLIM5, RGS4
NMDA and glutamate-related (glutamate pathway)	DAO, DAOA, , **DTNBP1** (**Dysbindin**), GRIA1(works on Axon guidance and neurite outgrowth), GRID1, GRIN1, GRIN2A, GRIN2B, GRIK4, GRM3, GRM4, GRM7, NOS1, NOSIAP, SYN3(synapsin-III)
Dopaminergic/Serotonergic	**COMT**, **DRD2**, **DRD3**, HTR2A, HTR5A, HTR6, SLC6A3, SLC6A4, SLC18A1, SLC18A2, **MAOA**, TH
Circadian control	CLOCK, TIMELESS, PER3
Cytokines signaling and immune-related	CSF2RB, IL1B (Interleukins), IL1RN, TNFA (Tumor Necrosis Factor)
Oxidative and other stress: Glutathione: Plays an important role in the detoxification of dopamine/catecholamine derived quinine	ND4, NDUFV2
Methionine and homocysteine metabolism	MTHFR, MTHFD, MTR
Endoplasmic reticulum stress	XBP1
Miscellaneous	APOE, BRD1, CHRNA7, DISC1 (Disrupted in schizophrenia 1, Involved in neurite outgrowth and cortical development), DPYSL2, GPR50, MLC1, PPP3CC (Calcineurin), SYNGR1, YWHAH (works on serotonin receptors)

Chromosome 22q11 deletion syndrome is also known as velocardiofacial syndrome, DiGeorge syndrome, and Shprintzen syndrome. Overall, 1% to 2% of individuals with schizophrenia have 22q11 deletion syndrome. This is medically significant because a range of associated conditions exists. Those conditions include cardiac defects,

Causes of Schizophrenia

immune system dysfunction, platelet abnormalities, and hypocalcemia. Clinical features of 22q11 deletion syndrome in individuals with schizophrenia or first-episode psychosis include the following:

- Childhood learning difficulties, developmental delay, articulation disorder.
- Palatal features, such as hypernasal speech, high arched palate, or history of cleft palate.
- A history of congenital cardiac abnormalities.
- Cranio-facial abnormalities.
- Other physical congenital abnormalities, including abnormal fingers, high arches, and scoliosis.
- A history of recurrent ear infections or hearing loss may also be relevant.

A person who has 22q11 deletion syndrome may be advised to seek genetic counseling.

A person who has 22q11 deletion syndrome may be advised to seek genetic counseling.

At this point, there is a tremendous quantity of research on the relation of genetics and schizophrenia. Most of it has not been replicated; therefore, we cannot yet say that genetic changes are directly responsible for schizophrenia. One or many abnormal genes together may be acting during different stages of the life of an individual. The brain may have different levels of sensitivity during the life span.

- In the fetal and the early years phase, some brain structures may develop abnormally with no evident clinical symptom.
- During adolescence, the connections between neurons may change anatomically or functionally. Because of the change, a psychotic process may appear spontaneously or due to the interaction with an environmental factor.

- Later on, there may be less brain plasticity in the aging brain.

Schizophrenia is now thought as a **neurodevelopmental** disorder.

Some genes may give rise to traits associated with schizophrenia but not the disease itself. The existence of multiple genes predisposing for schizophrenia may help explain the variability of symptoms across individuals.

Neurodevelop-mental

Happening during the growth and formation of different structures of the brain.

27. So is genetic testing worth doing for schizophrenia? Is the research on this making headway?

As of today it is unlikely that a specific genetic testing will be available in the foreseeable future to detect whether a child has inherited the risk for schizophrenia. There are no genetic tests yet that are sensitive enough or specific enough to do this. As with many other diseases, there are roughly three hypotheses regarding the genetic cause of a disease.

1. One specific single gene is abnormal and produces schizophrenia. It is a disease of one specific gene. No other genes are involved and an abnormality in a different gene would not produce schizophrenia. (Monogenic single major locus model).

2. A single abnormality in one of many genes could produce schizophrenia. That is, schizophrenia is many different diseases each due to an abnormality of a different gene. Thus sometimes the abnormality is transmitted to the offspring (either recessively or dominantly) or is not transmitted at all (Distinct heterogeneity model).

Causes of Schizophrenia

3. Multiple genes with abnormalities interact externally or environmentally and combine their effects to produce the disease. Thus, sometimes it is inherited and sometimes not. There may be a certain number or severity of the abnormality required before the disease occurs (Multifactorial-polygenic threshold model).

None of these models has been clearly shown to be the correct one. In fact, all three models may occur in different patients or families. This makes genetic testing quite tricky.

The hope of the field of pharmacogenomics and pharmacogenetics is to be able to tailor treatment of particular diseases to each individual's particular genetic make-up rather than using the "one size fits all" drugs now being used. Although exciting, this field is still in its infancy.

Research is continuing to better understand the disease, the genetics and the biological pathways and markers involved. The development of better treatments, in particular new and more specific medications, will be easier if clear genetic or environmental causes are identified. Until then, though, much of the pharmaceutical research will focus on the development of better molecules in the families of drugs that are known to work in order to find safer and more effective treatments. This work is based on clinical clues rather than genetics.

Another aim is to develop medicines that can be given at the first stages of the disease to prevent further deterioration.

The hope of the field of pharmacogenomics and pharmacogenetics is to be able to tailor treatment of particular diseases to each individual's particular genetic make-up rather than using the "one size fits all" drugs now being used. Although exciting, this field is still in its infancy.

28. We have one child with schizophrenia. Should we go and see a genetic counselor?

Yes. This is often very useful and wise.

Counseling helps with the complex and fast moving field of genetics. It helps families to understand the nature of the disease and what options there might be for prevention and testing, the risk of recurrence and the implications for other family members.

Genetic counseling is nondirective, nonjudgmental and supports people in reaching their own decisions. No two patients are the same and a diagnosis can have a very different meaning to different people.

Most people are referred to a genetics counselor by their physician following a diagnosis. In the case of schizophrenia, as there is no genetic testing available, a good history of the mental illnesses in the family will be needed for the **geneticist** to evaluate the risks. The counselor may be able also to give recommendations on how to reduce the risks by better pregnancy planning, avoiding stress during the pregnancy, and getting involved during the pregnancy and after the birth of the child in activities that will maximize the child's mental health.

29. What does it mean when doctors talk about chemical imbalance?

The current state of psychiatric and neurologic thinking is that schizophrenia, as well as many other psychiatric diseases, may be due to abnormalities, imbalances, excesses, or shortages of chemicals in the brain or elsewhere.

Geneticists
Scientists who study the inheritance of traits in humans, animals, or plants.

The current state of psychiatric and neurologic thinking is that schizophrenia, as well as many other psychiatric diseases, may be due to abnormalities, imbalances, excesses or shortages of chemicals in the brain or elsewhere.

Causes of Schizophrenia

First, a brief word about neurotransmitters and receptors: A neurotransmitter is a chemical that carries nerve impulses across the fluid filled space between nerve cells. This chemical carries the impulse from one nerve cell to the next in the brain, down the spinal cord and to the distant parts of the body. Nerve cells in fact do not always touch each other. In order to send information from one nerve to the next, chemicals are released by the sending nerve, to the next nerve. There, they attach to specific or specialized receptors that are equipped to receive the message on the surface of the receiving nerve cell. Such chemicals include serotonin, **acetylcholine**, glutamate, **GABA, norepinephrine**, and dopamine. There are many others.

Much of the work in psychopharmacology (the drug treatment of psychiatric disease) is now aimed at neurotransmitters and their receptors.

Neurotransmitters: The Dopamine Hypothesis

The dopamine hypothesis emerged in the 1950s, as a result of the clinical discovery that a class of medications called the phenothiazines was able to control the positive symptoms (hallucinations, delusions) of schizophrenia. Studies on the mechanism of these drugs showed that they function by blocking the functioning of molecules called *dopamine D2 receptors*, which sit on the surface of certain nerve cells and convey dopamine's signals to the cells.

At the same time, amphetamine, which was known to induce hallucinations and delusions in habitual abusers, was found to stimulate dopamine release in the brain.

These two findings led to the dopamine theory, which is that most symptoms of schizophrenia are due to

Acetylcholine

A neurotransmitter in both the peripheral nervous system (PNS) and central nervous system (CNS).

GABA

A neurotransmitter whose role is to inhibit the flow of nerve signals by blocking the release of other neurotransmitters.

Norepinephrine

A neurotransmitter that regulates arousal, sleep, blood pressure and may produce anxiety.

excess dopamine release in certain important brain regions. There may be too many receptors (increased density) or increased sensitivity of the receptors or both.

Specifically in schizophrenia, it is felt that the negative (apathy, poverty of speech, withdrawal) and cognitive symptoms may originate from *reduced* dopamine levels in certain parts of the brain, such as the frontal lobes (thought to regulate abstract thinking), and *increased* dopamine in other parts of the brain, such as the limbic system (thought to regulate emotions). This is the imbalance portion of the hypothesis.

Neurotransmitters: The Glutamate Hypothesis

A second hypothesis revolves around the neurotransmitter glutamate and suggests that abnormally low activity may produce the symptoms.

This hypothesis came about when it was noticed that some patients who received the anesthetic phencyclidine (PCP), which is a glutamate antagonist, developed hallucinations. Further experimental work showed that volunteers given lower doses of PCP developed not just hallucinations but also thought disorders and psychotic symptoms. These lasted a few hours and disappeared.

Next, work was done on glutamate receptors. Various subunits of the glutamate receptors, called NMDA receptors, were identified. NMDA receptors amplify neural signals and help the brain respond to some messages and ignore others, facilitating attention. People with schizophrenia respond differently to sounds than people without the disease, which implies that their brain circuits (relying on NMDA receptors) are different. Remember the abnormal evoked responses on the EEG discussed in question 21? Further work suggests that reduced activity in these NMDA receptors may produce the symptoms of schizophrenia as the brain processes information abnormally.

If reduced NMDA receptor activity produces schizophrenia's symptoms, what then causes this reduction? It is unclear. Fewer NMDA receptors? An abnormal glutamate release? An abnormal NMDA activity?

Short-term trials with agents known to stimulate NMDA receptors have produced encouraging results, adding support to the glutamate hypothesis. If proved effective, these agents will become the first entirely new class of medicines developed specifically to target the negative and cognitive symptoms of schizophrenia.

Neurotransmitters: The Serotonin Hypothesis

The serotonin (5-HT) hypothesis of schizophrenia arose from studies on interactions between the hallucinogenic drug LSD (D-lysergic acid diethylamide) and serotonin (5-HT) in peripheral systems. The actions of the hallucinogens have been shown to be mediated by particular receptors called 5-HT (2A) receptors found in two brain regions (the locus coeruleus and the **cerebral cortex**).

Cerebral cortex

Most superficial part of the brain, responsible for higher level of thought processes like language, and information processing.

These neurotransmitter hypotheses represent a possible explanation for (at least) some cases of schizophrenia. The development of specific drugs to increase or decrease neurotransmitter activity in the specific brain locations involved continues and represents an exciting area of research.

Polyunsaturated Fatty Acids (PUFA)

Another imbalance hypothesis relates to the finding that dietary supplementation with certain fatty acids improved some symptoms of schizophrenia. Since fatty acids are required for healthy cell membranes in the brain it was suggested that the problem here may be in abnormal absorption or metabolism of fatty acids. Further, abnormal nerve cell membranes in the brain might produce receptor problems.

An excellent review by the Cochrane Collaboration of published studies suggested that one particular type of fatty acid, ethyl eicosapentaenoic acid (an omega-3 EFA) may produce beneficial effects though the results were not conclusive. Scientists are continuing their research.

30. Who should do the evaluation of my child?

It is important that a psychiatrist (preferably a child psychiatrist) does the first evaluation. This physician will ask many questions concerning the child and the family. For example:

- Questions about the mother's pregnancy, labor and delivery.
- Early childhood development, milestones.
- Medical and psychiatric history of the child. General medical causes of psychotic symptoms should be ruled out. Some of those causes might include acute intoxication, delirium, central nervous system lesions, tumors or infections, metabolic disorders, drugs, and seizure disorders.
- Questions about the medical and psychiatric history of the family members and the extended family members.
- Age and nature of the symptoms at onset.

An excellent review by the Cochrane Collaboration of published studies suggested that one particular type of fatty acid, ethyl eicosapen-taenoic acid (an omega-3 EFA) may produce beneficial effects though the results were not conclusive.

Causes of Schizophrenia

The psychiatric evaluation will include the assessment of any thought disturbance, hallucinations, delusions, cognition level, any negative symptoms (which have a strong prognostic value), symptoms of depression or mania, any suicidal or homicidal ideations, level of judgment, insight, level of impulse control, memory status, pattern of communication, age-appropriate developmental level, and social deficits.

A full physical examination is needed to look for any associated medical conditions.

The doctor will search for any neurological symptoms and may ask for a neurological consultation, which may include EEG and CAT scan of the brain. A full physical examination is needed to look for any associated medical conditions. Evaluation of potential substance abuse (particularly in adolescents). Blood and urine tests will be ordered and might include a drug screening.

It is only after these tests are completed that a psychological examination might be ordered to have a more precise evaluation of:

- Intellectual level (IQ)
- Projective testing which will provide information about the severity of the psychotic thinking
- Assessment of communication skills
- Assessment of adaptive functions

Sometimes genetic testing may be ordered.

31. What laboratory tests are done and what could they show?

Laboratory studies are performed for the differential diagnosis.

- Toxicology screens may be needed if there is a possibility of substance abuse.
- Liver function tests, copper and ceruloplasmin levels may be ordered to eliminate Wilson disease, which may produce liver and psychiatric problems.
- Porphobilinogen for the diagnosis of porphyria.
- Human immunodeficiency virus (HIV) test, Venereal Disease Research Laboratory (VDRL) testing, or heavy metal screening (lead levels) may be done.

Prior to starting and during treatment with certain medications, routine laboratory studies are needed:

- Antipsychotic medications may cause abnormalities in blood and liver functions. Glucose and lipid abnormalities will need to be monitored.
- Clozapine may cause severe leucopenia and regular blood tests are needed.
- Thyroid and renal functions are required prior to starting lithium.

If the child has mental retardation or abnormal features, a genetic assessment may be needed (for example: in the 22q11 deletion syndrome, or velocardiofacial syndrome).

If the child has mental retardation or abnormal features, a genetic assessment may be needed (for example: in the 22q11 deletion syndrome, or velocardiofacial syndrome).

32. What does an electroencephalogram (EEG) show?

Various studies have been done looking at the use of EEGs in schizophrenic children. Abnormal findings, such as "spike and wave" changes are seen in around 50% of the children studied, but by no means in all of them. Thus, the use of EEGs cannot be used alone to make the diagnosis.

An EEG may be useful if episodic symptoms are present in a child with psychosis. This may help in making the diagnosis of an associated seizure disorder.

An EEG may be useful if episodic symptoms are present in a child with psychosis. This may help in making the diagnosis of an associated seizure disorder.

Psychotic symptoms can occur in epilepsy, in particular with temporal and frontal lobe partial seizures. Ambulatory electroencephalogram monitoring may be required. This technique means that the child can go about his or her daily business while wearing the apparatus rather than having to stay in a medical facility. The ambulatory device registers the brain waves over an extended period of time during the day and the night.

In children who receive clozapine, an EEG may be necessary due to the increased risk of seizures associated with this medication.

Gray matter

The brownish-gray nerve tissue of the brain and spinal cord that contains the nerve cells.

White matter

Whitish brain and spinal cord tissue composed mostly of nerve fibers and its shiny protective coat called myelin.

Ventricles

As this term applies to the brain, the spaces connecting throughout the brain that provide a system for the circulation of the fluid present in the brain called cerebrospinal fluid.

33. What do radiology tests like scans show?

Studies in adolescent schizophrenia showed findings similar to those in adult schizophrenia. MRIs in adolescent schizophrenia have shown a consistent pattern of decreased cerebral (brain) volume, and ventricular dilatation. There is relative **gray matter** reduction with **white matter** sparing. The most common finding with CAT (CT) imaging in first-episode psychosis is enlargement of the **ventricles** and cortical sulci (fissures on the surface of the brain) which may be present in 30% to 40% of patients.

The total cerebral volume is correlated with negative symptoms. Radiological studies over time may provide direct evidence of progressive brain changes after the beginning of the psychotic process.

Rare neurodegenerative disorders that can mimic schizophrenia will be differentiated with the use of MRI:

- Wilson's disease will show low density areas in the **basal ganglia** together with cortical atrophy and ventricular dilatation.
- Metachromatic leukodystrophy will show frontal and occipital white matter destruction and demyelination.

Basal ganglia

A group of neurons inside the brain that has an important role in the control of movements and behaviors.

Causes of Schizophrenia

PART FOUR

Differential Diagnosis

What is the difference between schizophreniform
disorder and schizophrenia?

My son hears voices but the psychiatrist says
it is not schizophrenia. Why?

My son has an imaginary friend. Will he become
schizophrenic?

More . . .

34. My child seems to have multiple personalities. He talks to different people using different voices. Sometimes he is an angel and does what he is supposed to do and sometimes he acts like a monster. What is going on here? What does this mean?

The existence of multiple personalities within an individual is called dissociative identity disorder (DID). Prior to the publication of the DSM-IV, it was termed multiple personality disorder (MPD). DID is a controversial diagnosis. It is sometimes called split personality. It is assumed to be a mental disorder, originating in children who are stressed or abused, especially sexually abused. DID is characterized by changes in consciousness, identity, memory, motor behavior, or environmental awareness. Schizophrenia is in the differential diagnosis because patients often hear voices; the difference in DID is that they hear voices within their heads, not from outside.

Although many people may think of schizophrenia as a patient having multiple personalities, this is actually not the case.

Although many people may think of schizophrenia as a patient having multiple personalities, this is actually not the case. As noted above, a patient with true multiple personalities probably does not have schizophrenia. The psychiatrist is usually able to make the distinction between the two diseases. Multiple Personality Disorder is unusual in younger patients.

35. What is the difference between psychosis and schizophrenia?

Psychosis is a symptom of mental illness, but it is not a mental illness in its own right. Psychosis (or psychotic thinking or psychotic symptoms) means a mental state or condition characterized by loss of contact with reality. There may also be hallucinations and delusions.

Psychosis is a hallmark of schizophrenia but the presence of psychosis does not automatically mean schizophrenia. Psychosis can occur in people who do or do not have other mental illnesses. The symptoms may be due to an adverse drug reaction, extreme stress, a seizure disorder, sleep deprivation, brain infections or tumors and other medical or psychiatric illnesses.

People with schizophrenia often experience psychosis, as well as people with bipolar disorder, severe depression, delirium, or substance abuse. These patients can also have long periods without psychosis.

Psychosis is a hallmark of schizophrenia but the presence of psychosis does not automatically mean schizophrenia.

36. What is the difference between schizophreniform disorder and schizophrenia?

The difference between these terms is the duration of the symptom period (**Table 4**). The symptoms of both are the same. However, in **schizophreniform** disorders, the symptoms usually last from 1 to 6 months and then disappear. In schizophrenia the symptoms last more than 6 months. About half of those diagnosed with schizophreniform disorder are later diagnosed with schizophrenia. The diagnosis of schizophrenia generally cannot be made unless the symptoms are present for more than 6 months.

Schizophreniform

Having the symptoms of schizophrenia, but too early in the course of illness to tell whether the symptoms are of a schizophrenia illness.

Table 4 Duration of Symptoms & Diagnosis

Less than 1 month: Brief psychotic disorder
>1 month, <6 months: Schizophreniform disorder
Greater than 6 months: Schizophrenia

Differential Diagnosis

37. If you can have a psychotic process in mood disorders, how do you know the difference between a mood disorder and schizophrenia?

Broadly speaking, there are two types of psychiatric disorders. There are the psychotic disorders, such as schizophrenia, and the mood disorders, such as depression. The problems occur when symptoms of one class of disorders are seen in the other. Thus, the differentiation and diagnosis can be very difficult because a mood disturbance can be seen also in schizophrenia to some degree and some psychotic symptoms may be seen in mood disorders.

1. Depression with psychotic features.

    A major depressive episode, where the patient whose mood is depressed experiences psychotic symptoms such as delusions or hallucinations. These are most commonly mood-congruent and the contents of the thoughts have depressive themes, paralleling the mood. The symptoms persist for at least 2 weeks. The episode may be either single or recurrent. Diagnosis in children or adolescents may be delayed or missed if the symptoms are thought to be normal moodiness. The child's mood may be more irritable than depressed.

    In children, schizophrenia may start by looking like severe depression (irritability, withdrawal from social contacts, decline in academic performance, poor concentration, sleeping too much or too little) and the diagnosis may be missed at that point, particularly when the child denies anything is wrong. Children may deny that anything is wrong because they do not want to tell or they do not recognize that there are hallucinations or mild delusions.

2. Bipolar depression or manic-depressive disorder.

This is a category of mood disorders defined by the presence of one or more episodes of abnormally elevated mood, referred to as mania or hypomania. The features of mania are rapid speech and rapid thoughts, and risky behaviors. If the symptoms are milder then it is considered hypomania. Individuals who experience **manic** episodes also commonly experience depressive episodes, or mixed episodes in which features of both mania and depression are present at the same time. These episodes are normally separated by periods of normal mood, but in some patients, depression and mania may rapidly alternate, which is called *rapid cycling*. Manic episodes can sometimes lead to psychotic symptoms such as delusions and hallucinations.

Children with bipolar disorder do not often meet the strict DSM-IV definition, and tend to have rapid-cycling or mixed-cycling patterns.

Thus children with bipolar disorders may have some elements of psychosis but eventually the correct diagnosis of mood disorder is able to be made.

3. Schizoaffective disorder.

This is a condition where symptoms of a mood disorder (depression, mania, or both) and symptoms of schizophrenia are both present. There is a baseline of psychosis in addition to which mood episodes occur.

The onset of schizoaffective disorder is most frequent during late adolescence and early adulthood, although, more rarely, it can be diagnosed in childhood. Psychiatrists may make the diagnosis of schizophrenia at one point and the diagnosis of schizoaffective disorder or bipolar disorder at another

Manic

Feeling excessively elated and cheery with very fast speech and thoughts.

The onset of schizoaffective disorder is most frequent during late adolescence and early adulthood, although, more rarely, it can be diagnosed in childhood.

Differential Diagnosis

point of the disease as the symptoms become clearer over time.

There may be a biologic continuum between all these diagnoses. Unlike medical diseases where objective biologic or radiologic tests can be done to make a clear diagnosis (e.g., a blood test shows iron deficiency anemia) psychiatric diagnosis relies primarily on clinical examination and, occasionally, on psychology testing which are more subjective than objective. It is hoped that when objective tests are developed that diagnosis will become clearer and easier.

Diagnostic confusion can occur because the positive symptoms of psychosis can be seen in mood disorders (sometimes called affective psychosis). The presence of negative symptoms and an insidious onset are the best predictors of adolescent schizophrenia while early (in less than 6 months) and complete remission of symptoms are the best predictors of a diagnosis of a mood disorder.

38. My son hears voices but the psychiatrist says it is not schizophrenia. Why?

Psychotic experiences may be present in 5% to 20% of the general population. Many of these people will have no mental illnesses, but some will have schizophrenia in the future and some will have other mental disorders.

Sometimes, hearing voices is very benign. This is frequent when people are falling asleep (they are called hypnagogic hallucinations) or when people are just waking up (hypnopompic hallucinations).

Children sometimes hear their name being called or hear a sound but this is not a serious symptom if infrequent. However, when such symptoms appear, the child should be followed to see if the voices disappear or if other symptoms appear.

39. My son has an imaginary friend. Will he become schizophrenic?

Imaginary friends (people or animals) are pretend characters often created by children—usually around the age of 3 or 4 years. Imaginary friends function as a protector or a buddy when they are engaged by the child in play activity. Imaginary friends may exist for the child into adolescence and sometimes adulthood. They often have elaborate personalities. They may seem very real but children understand that their imaginary friends are not real. They may serve a very positive purpose for the child by helping the child to deal with stresses. It is not a psychotic process. If your child plays happily with others and enjoys doing things with you and other children there is not likely to be any problem. If this is not the case, it will be helpful to have a look at what is going on in his life and think about ways to help him enjoy doing real things as well.

They may seem very real but children understand that their imaginary friends are not real.

40. My child is schizophrenic and his doctor says that he became catatonic. What does that mean?

Catatonia is relatively rare but can be seen in schizophrenia. The symptoms are either complete immobility and muteness (stupor) or extreme disorganization and excitability (catatonic excitement). It is a serious situation.

According to the DSM-IV, at least two of the following must be present:

- Motor immobility as evidenced by catalepsy (muscular rigidity and fixed posture, including waxy

Differential Diagnosis

flexibility, the tendency to maintain an immobile posture, the limbs tend to remain in whatever position they are placed) or stupor;

- Excessive motor activity (purposeless, not influenced by external stimuli);
- Extreme negativism (motiveless resistance to all instructions or maintenance of a rigid posture against attempts to move the limbs) or mutism;
- Peculiarities of movement as evidenced by posturing, stereotyped movements, mannerisms, or grimacing;
- Echolalia (the repetition of vocalizations made by another person) or echopraxia (involuntary repetition or imitation of the observed movements of another person).

Catatonia is associated with psychiatric conditions such as schizophrenia (catatonic type) and bipolar disorder. It may also be seen in many medical disorders including infections (such as encephalitis), strokes and metabolic disturbances. It has some similarity to conditions such as **neuroleptic** malignant syndrome that we will discuss later.

Neuroleptic

Any medication that when given to animals will cause catalepsy.

From Tony, Vicky's 20-year-old brother:

Vicky, my 16-year-old sister, started acting really strange at home when I was visiting from school during the Christmas break. It looked like she stopped cleaning herself, taking showers—even not wiping herself after going to the toilet. She stopped coming out of her room for meals, and wouldn't speak with me or our brother Bob or mom or dad. She seemed to be in her own world, doing nothing. Last Saturday (5 days ago) she stopped eating and drinking completely and stayed in bed. She wouldn't talk to us and didn't even seem to hear us when we spoke to her. If we tried to get her out of bed, it was like dead weight. She wouldn't move. We knew she wasn't dead because she was breathing and her eyes moved. Dad called our doctor who said to call an ambulance to bring her to the hospital where they admitted her to the psych unit. She wouldn't take the medicine in her mouth or eat or drink so they had to start an IV but then they had to transfer her to the intensive care unit because they said she was so dry her heart was beating funny. I guess they fed her by vein and gave her the medicine that way because she sort of woke up the next day. By Tuesday she was talking a little to me and my brother Bob when we went to see her. I had to go back to school but Dad called me to tell me she's better now and out of the ICU but still in the hospital. She's taking the pills by mouth and they hope she can go home next week. This is very scary and sad and I hope Bob and I don't become like that.

PART FIVE

Treatment of Schizophrenia: Medications

Can schizophrenia be treated without
medication in children?

If my child is to take medications, are
there questions to ask the doctor?

Are there any special precautions that we
should take when our child is put on
antipsychotic medications?

More . . .

41. What are the consequences if my child with schizophrenia is not treated? After all, the problems may go away.

Schizophrenia does not go away. Symptoms may go up and down but they do not really go away.

Schizophrenia does not go away. Symptoms may go up and down but they do not really go away. The consequences of nontreatment can be devastating, both in childhood and in adulthood.

In childhood, as you are probably aware, problems occur in the family setting, in the school setting, in personal interactions, all of which can be terrible for both the child and the family.

In adulthood, one may see:

- Homelessness
- Episodes of violence. One study showed a 50% reduction in the rate of violence in schizophrenics treated for their illness.
- Incarcerations, often as a result of the violence.
- Victimization. Crimes against individuals with severe psychiatric disorders are common and often not reported to the police.
- Suicide. Suicide is the number one cause of premature death among people with schizophrenia, with an estimated 10% to 13% killing themselves. These suicide rates are striking when compared to the general population where the rate is approximately 1%.
- Monetary costs. The problems cited above produce monetary costs both to society but also to the individual in terms of costs relating to loss of work, hospitalizations, and legal charges if they exist.
- The largest cost, of course, is intangible and that is the affect on the family.

People with schizophrenia are often unable to contribute economically to society and many require costly services from society for the rest of their lives. This is bad for both the individual and society.

Treatment needs to be individualized to the needs of the child to make it as acceptable and nontraumatic as possible. The evaluation is usually done by the school system, the parents and the medical team and sometimes community agencies. Treating youth with Early Onset Schizophrenia (EOS) often requires a continuum of services and treatment providers. In addition to psychopharmacology management and **psychotherapy**, many of these youths need extensive case management and community support services. Such services may include crisis intervention, family support programs, and in-home services.

From a mother:

Shakirah, my 11-year-old, started telling me last week that she is afraid coming home from school when she sees a little girl covered with blood standing on the corner of 11th Street, right in front of the school. This little girl was always the same and was making gestures as if she wanted Shakirah to come with her. Shakirah said no one else saw this girl because she would be invisible to them. This morning her home room teacher called me because she thought a girl with blood was coming for her. They told me to take her home and see our doctor right away. I made an appointment for 3 pm today.

42. What is the rationale for medications? Will it be the only treatment?

Childhood-onset schizophrenia is a severe and chronic medical and neurological disease which requires early and aggressive treatment with an antipsychotic medication.

Treating youth with EOS often requires a continuum of services and treatment providers.

Psychotherapy
The treatment of mental or emotional problems by psychological means.

Treatment of Schizophrenia: Medications

Most antipsychotic medications are divided into two types.

- Typical, or first-generation, antipsychotics are all high-affinity antagonists of dopamine D2 receptors. Their basic therapeutic effect is that they bind tightly and fairly specifically to dopamine receptors.
- **Atypical**, or second-generation, antipsychotics attach to dopamine D2 receptors and other receptors. They have become the treatment of choice in the US.

Currently all effective antipsychotic medications block the D2 dopamine receptor, a specialized protein which dopamine attaches to in the brain cells. Blockade of the D2 receptor appears to be a necessary condition for antipsychotic response. Blockade of other brain receptors, like, the serotonin 2 receptor, or alterations of other brain chemicals such as GABA, glutamate, and neurotensin (an endogenous neurotransmitter that has associations with the dopamine neurotransmitter system) may also be a mechanism of action of antipsychotic drugs.

General Principles of Treatment

Pharmacotherapy with antipsychotic medications is an essential component.

- Medications must be individualized patient by patient. One size does not fit all.
- Patients with a first episode of psychosis usually require a lower dosage.
- Simple medication regimens, such as once-daily dosing, promote adherence to treatment.
- Dosages should be maintained within the recommended range. Reasons for going outside the range need to be justified.

Atypical
One of the second-generation antipsychotic medications.

Pharmacotherapy
Treatment of disease through the use of drugs.

Medications must be individualized patient by patient. One size does not fit all.

- There is no evidence supporting the use of more than one antipsychotic drug simultaneously.
- Psychosocial interventions work synergistically with medication to optimize treatment adherence.
- Patients and families, where possible, must be involved in decisions and choices for pharmacotherapy. They must be provided with information on the risks and benefits of both taking and not taking medications.

Treatment can vary depending upon the phase of the disease. This classification (acute and chronic is now somewhat dated)

In the acute phase:
- Psychoeducation is of primary importance and it is also an ongoing process. Childhood-onset schizophrenia is a family issue. Everyone in the family has to be educated and learn as much as possible about schizophrenia, which is severe, chronic, debilitating, very difficult to treat, disruptive and may produce significant disability and residual psychotic symptoms.
- Medications. Typical and atypical antipsychotics are discussed elsewhere in the book.
- Psychotherapy. **Cognitive behavioral therapy** can help the child with schizophrenia to cope with the symptoms of the disease. Other types of psychotherapy may be useful to the child to deal with life stressors, to understand the illness, to comply with treatment, to improve self-esteem and to learn how to better socialize. **Family therapy** may also be necessary to help family members to deal with the patient in the home setting, to navigate through the multiple government, school, and social agencies involved with therapy and assistance.

Cognitive behavioral therapy

This is a brief form of psychotherapy based on the principle that the way one thinks about something causes actions.

Family therapy

Any of several therapeutic approaches in which a family is treated as a whole.

In the chronic phase:

- Medication maintenance to improve outcome and prevent relapses.
- Medication follow up to minimize drug side effects.
- Supportive individual or group therapies.
- Family therapy as needed.
- Multifamily groups for support.
- Guiding education and rehabilitation.

A more modern approach is to divide schizophrenia into more specific phases.

- Prodromal phase—the early period of deteriorating function without the full blown disease being present.
- Psychotic phase—the classic symptoms are now present.
- Recovery phase—the active psychosis begins to remit but there are still some ongoing psychotic symptoms. This phase may also be associated with confusion, disorganization.
- Residual phase—positive psychotic symptoms are minimal, but ongoing negative symptoms, such as social withdrawal, apathy, amotivation, and flat affect, are frequent.
- Chronic phase impairment—persistent symptoms that have not responded adequately to treatment remain.

43. Can schizophrenia be treated without medication in children?

Absolutely not. People with schizophrenia who take medications will definitely relapse back to psychosis if they stop their medications. The relapse may not occur for several weeks or a few months. This period of doing well after stopping antipsychotic drugs may give

People with schizophrenia who take medications will definitely relapse back to psychosis if they stop their medications.

the false impression that the patient can do well without medications. However, psychosis will return and that is a serious matter because psychosis is associated with loss of brain tissue. With every psychotic relapse, the brain deteriorates more. In addition, it may be harder to induce a remission after a relapse due to medication being stopped.

With every psychotic relapse, the brain deteriorates more.

Nonadherence to medications is common in schizophrenia for many reasons.

1. Not realizing that one has an illness. This may apply to the child and to the parents;
2. Lack of motivation, which is one of the deficit symptoms in schizophrenia;
3. Memory difficulties;
4. Alcohol and drug abuse, which impair judgment about the need to take one's medicine;
5. Fear of side effects.

Although it may be difficult, parents should put in place a mechanism to ensure that their child takes his or her medications as prescribed. This can be challenging but is absolutely necessary.

44. Will my child respond differently from adults to the medication?

Children are not just small adults. They may respond in a different way to medications than adults do.

Children often metabolize and eliminate drugs more quickly than adults. This means that children may have to be given higher doses ("adult-size" doses) in order to get good therapeutic effects. On the other hand, an adult dose in some children would be too much and could be an overdose. In addition, each person may respond differently to the same dose of a drug, so doses must be tailored to the individual patient. The dose used of any drug should be the smallest dose that effectively treats your child's symptoms.

At different ages, a child can respond differently to the same dose of a drug because the central nervous system is at different stages of development.

At different ages, a child can respond differently to the same dose of a drug because the central nervous system is at different stages of development. This is not usually true for adults whose development has reached maturity. No two children respond to antipsychotic medication in the same way. Sometimes a child will not respond to any medication and sometimes a child will respond differently to each of the antipsychotic medications. There is no way to predict how a child will respond to a particular drug. The only way to know is to try the drug. Trials of medications should last at least 4 to 6 weeks, though sometimes a trial for as long as 6 months may be useful if there is some positive response to the medication. Of course, there should be regular monitoring by the treating physician.

The occurrence of side effects varies markedly from one medication to another as well as from one child to another. For example, adolescents have a higher risk than adults of abnormal side effects to certain antipsychotic drugs. Some of those side effects are **dystonic** reactions such as abnormal muscle tension or tone. If the side effects are a problem, reducing the dose of the medication is often sufficient. Alternatively, stopping this drug and switching to another medication may give equal benefits with fewer side effects.

Dystonic
A neurological movement disorder in which sustained muscle contractions cause twisting or abnormal postures.

45. What first-generation, typical antipsychotic (FGA) medications are used?

This refers to the class of dopamine D2 receptors antagonists. As a group these drugs, which are the earliest antipsychotics (or neuroleptics or major **tranquilizers**) discovered, have good therapeutic effects but also high rate of unwanted side effects. Generally the doses are higher in adolescents than in children and higher in the acute phase of the illness than in the maintenance phase (**Table 5** and **Table 6**).

Tranquilizers
Any drug that is used to calm or pacify an anxious and/or agitated person.

46. What second (SGA) and third generation (TGA) atypical antipsychotic medications are used?

These newer drugs have a lower-affinity for D2 receptors and greater affinity for other neuroreceptors and for that reason, different side effects.

47. What are the side effects of antipsychotic medications?

Because schizophrenia is chronic and needs long-term treatment, the monitoring of drug side effects is very important. The choice of the antipsychotic will also be determined by considering, in advance, the possible risks of the medicines.

All antipsychotics can have side effects—as can all drugs. As noted above, the typical drugs have, among others, **extrapyramidal** side effects while the atypicals often have metabolic complications. The role of the physician is to monitor them and to minimize them as much as possible. As noted above, other than broad comments about the typicals and atypicals, it is not possible to predict which side effects will or might occur in a particular patient.

Extrapyramidal
The extrapyramidal system is a neural network located in the brain that is part of the motor system involved in the coordination of movement.

Treatment of Schizophrenia: Medications

Table 5   Drugs Used in Childhood Schizophrenia

Generic Name	Trade Name	Availability	Use in Children	FDA Approval	Usual Dose Needed
Haloperidol	Haldol	Tablets: 0.5 mg, 1 mg, 2 mg, 5 mg, 10 mg, 20 mg Oral solution: 1 mg/ml, 2 mg/ml Injection: 5 mg/ml	Not recommended in children under 3 Toxic doses reported in children <6 years of age reported as: 0.15 mg/kg	Federal Drug Administration (FDA) approved in adult schizophrenia but not in children schizophrenia	Children: 1–4 mg/day Adolescents: 2–10 mg/day
	Haldol Decanoate	Injection (depot given q 4 weeks): 50 mg/ml, 100 mg/ml			Children: 15–50 mg q 4 weeks Adolescents: 50–100 mg q 4 weeks
Pimozide	Orap	Tablets: 2 mg, 4 mg	Limited data in children under 12	Not FDA approved	Usual dose: 1–5 mg/day
Chlorpromazine	Thorazine	Tablets: 10 mg, 25 mg, 50 mg, 100 mg, 200 mg Oral solution: 30 mg/ml, 100 mg/ml Oral syrup: 10 mg/5ml Injection: 25 mg/ml	Not recommended in children under 6 months Toxic doses in children <6 years of age reported as 15 mg/kg	Not FDA approved in children with schizophrenia	Children: 150–200 mg/day Adolescents: 225–375 mg/day

Fluphenazine	Prolixine	Tablets: 1 mg, 2.5 mg, 5 mg, 10 mg Oral solution: 2.5 mg/ml, 5 mg/ml Injection: 2.5 mg/ml	Safety and efficacy not established in children under age 12	Not FDA approved in children with schizophrenia	Chidren: 1.5–5 mg/day Adolescents: 2.5–10 mg/day
	Prolixin Decanoate	Injection (depot): 25 mg/ml	Depot form contre-indicated before age 12		
Perphenazine	Trilifon	Tablets: 2 mg, 4 mg, 8 mg, 16 mg Oral solution: 16 mg/5ml Injection: 5 mg/ml	Dosage recommendations for children over age 12	Not FDA approved in children with schizophrenia	Children: 6–12 mg/day Adolescents: 12–22 mg/day
Trifluoperazine	Stelazine	Tablets: 1 mg, 2 mg, 5 mg, 10 mg, Oral solution: 10 mg/ml Injection: 5 mg/ml	Dosage recommendations for children age 6–12	Not FDA approved for children with schizophrenia	Children: 2–10 mg/day Adolescents: 6–15 mg/day

(Continued)

Table 5 Drugs Used in Childhood Schizophrenia (Continued)

Generic Name	Trade Name	Availability	Use in Children	FDA Approval	Usual Dose Needed
Thioridazine	Mellaril	Tablets: 10 mg, 15 mg, 25 mg, 50 mg, 100 mg, 150 mg, 200 mg Oral solution: 30 mg/ml, 100 mg/ml	Dosage recommendations provided for children over age 2 Toxic doses in children <6 years of age reported as 1.4 mg/kg **Black box warning: cardiac toxicity**	Not FDA approved for children with schizophrenia	Children: 100–250 mg/day Adolescents: 225–325 mg/day
Thiothixene	Navane	Capsules: 1 mg, 2 mg, 5 mg, 10 mg, 20 mg Oral solution: 5 mg/ml Injection: 5 mg/ml		Not FDA approved in childhood schizophrenia	Children: 4–7 mg/day Adolescents: 4–20 mg/day
Loxapine	Loxitane	Capsules: 5 mg, 10 mg, 25 mg, 50 mg Oral solution: 25 mg/ml Injection: 50 mg/ml	Safety and efficacy not established in children	Not FDA approved in childhood schizophrenia	Usual dose: 50–100 mg/day

Table 6 Doses

Generic Name	Trade Name	Dosages/Forms	Comments	FDA Approval	Doses
Risperidone	Risperdal	Tablets: 0.25 mg, 0.5 mg, 1 mg, 2 mg, 3 mg, 4 mg, 5 mg Oral solution: 1mg/ml		Approved in child-hood schizophrenia for children >13 years old	Children: 1–2 mg/day Adolescents: 2.5–4 mg/day
	Risperdal M-Tab	Oral disintegrating tablets: 0.5 mg, 1 mg, 2 mg, 3 mg, 4 mg		As above	
	Risperdal Consta	Long-acting injection (q 2 weeks): 25 mg/vial, 37.5 mg/vial, 50 mg/vial		Approved only in adults	12.5–25 mg q 2 weeks
Clozapine	Clozaril	Tablets: 12.5 mg, 25mg, 50 mg, 100 mg, 200 mg	Safety and efficacy not established in children Used a lot in Europe	USA; max of 7 day prescription at a time Not FDA approved for children Strict blood monitoring	Start low (6.25 mg–12.5 mg) and increase gradually weekly. Children: 100–350 mg/day Adolescents: 225–450 mg/day
	Fazaclo ODT	Oral disintegrating tablets: 25 mg, 100 mg	As above	As above	As above

(Continued)

Table 6 Doses (Continued)

Generic Name	Trade Name	Dosages/Forms	Comments	FDA Approval	Doses
Olanzapine	Zyprexa	Tablets: 2.5 mg, 5 mg, 7.5 mg, 10 mg, 15 mg, 20 mg	Safety and efficacy not established in children	Not FDA approved for children schizophrenia	Children: 5–10 mg/day Adolescents: 10–15 mg/day
	Zyprexa Zydis	Oral dissolving tablets: 5 mg, 10 mg, 15 mg, 20 mg	As above	As above	As above
	Zyprexa intra-muscular	10 mg/vial	Contraindicated in children		
Quetiapine	Seroquel	Tablets: 25 mg, 50 mg, 100 mg, 200 mg, 300 mg, 400 mg	Safety and efficacy not established in children	Not FDA approved for children schizophrenia	Children: 150–400 mg/day Adolescents: 250–550 mg/day Given BID
	Seroquel XR				Given once a day
Ziprazidone	Geodon	Capsules: 20 mg, 40 mg, 60 mg, 80 mg Injection: 20 mg/ml	Safety and efficacy not established in children	Not FDA approved in children schizophrenia	Children: 40–100 mg/day Adolescents: 80–140 mg/day
Aripiprazole	Abilify	Tablets: 5 mg, 10 mg, 15 mg, 20 mg, 30 mg Oral solution: 1 mg/ml		Approved for childhood schizo-phrenia for chil-dren >13	Children: 5–15 mg/day Adolescents: 10–20 mg/day

Extrapyramidal Side Effects (EPS)

In COS, typical antipsychotics are associated with high levels of EPS and among the atypical antipsychotics, risperidone may be associated with more of these problems, especially at higher doses.

- This refers to abnormal dystonic (abnormal muscle tone) movements that arise very early in the treatment. They include muscle spasms, (usually mouth and face) with upward rotation of the eyes, stiffness in the neck, and protrusion of the tongue.
- Tardive **Dyskinesia**. This includes abnormal movements which can include lip smacking, tongue protrusion, continuous movements of the trunk and limbs. It is the most serious of the EPS as it does not always go away upon stopping the medication. It possibly occurs with long duration of treatment.
- Pseudoparkinsonism. This is characterized by muscle rigidity, bradykinesia (slowed or reduced voluntary movements) and tremor, similar to the classic Parkinson's Disease seen in older adults.

Dyskinesia
Difficulty in performing movements voluntarily.

Management of the EPS includes:

- Reducing the antipsychotic dose, if possible.
- Switching to an agent that has lower potential risk for EPS like quetiapine or olanzapine.
- In pseudoparkinsonism, use of **anticholinergic**s to counteract the side effects, allowing for continuing the medication.
- For tardive dyskinesia, switching to clozapine with intense blood monitoring, because of the risk of lowering white blood cells, or switching to an agent with lower risk of EPS.

Anticholinergic
An anticholinergic agent is a substance that blocks the neurotransmitter acetylcholine in the central and the peripheral nervous system.

Akathisia

Akathisia is an intense sensation of restlessness with a need for movement. It can be misinterpreted as worsening of the psychotic symptoms due to increased agitation. When the akathisia is interpreted as a worsening of the schizophrenia, the treating physician may actually increase the medicine that causes the akathisia, thereby worsening the problem. A high level of suspicion for this side effect must be maintained before attributing agitation to the COS. This is seen mostly with the typical antipsychotics but also with olanzapine, aripiprazole, and risperidone. It is seen the least with clozapine.

Management of akathisia:

- The usual initial response to this side effect is decreasing the medicine or switching to another one that may be less likely to produce this side effect.
- Use of the beta-blocker drug propanolol to slow the patient down a little.
- Less frequently, one of the benzodiazepine sedatives may be used such as lorazepam, more commonly known as Ativan. Sometimes an anticholinergic such as benztropine (Cogentin) is used.

Neuroleptic Malignant Syndrome

This is a rare but potentially life-threatening complication which arises in the early stages of the treatment. The signs include severe muscular rigidity, great variability of body temperature and blood pressure, as well as delirium. Laboratory findings include elevation of blood creatinine kinase (CPK) levels suggestive of muscle damage. In COS, atypical antipsychotics probably have a lower incidence and may produce a milder form of this syndrome when it does appear. Note that "neuroleptic" is a synonym for "antipsychotic drug."

Management of the neuroleptic malignant syndrome:

- The patient may need to be hospitalized.
- The antipsychotic drug should be stopped, even at the risk of worsening of the schizophrenia.
- Intensive supportive care including fluids (by vein if necessary), temperature control (e.g., acetaminophen).
- Where indicated, treatment with the drugs dantrolene and bromocriptine.

Seizures

All antipsychotic medications lower the seizure threshold and caution must be exercised with patients having a history of seizures. Seizures are reported to be rare with quetiapine (0.8%) and risperidone (0.3%).

Sedation

Sometimes sedation is difficult to differentiate from the negative symptoms of schizophrenia or from depression. In COS, sedation is seen with all antipsychotics, more frequently with clozapine (more than 50%), less frequently with olanzapine and quietapine (moderate sedation for both) and even less with risperidone and ziprazidone (mild sedation for both).

Management:

- Use as low a dose as possible.
- Encourage activities to keep the child moving.

Weight Gain

This is the focus of much interest now due to the increased awareness of the risks of childhood obesity. In a recent study, over a period of 8 weeks, children treated with olanzapine gained about 15 pounds, with

This is the focus of much interest now due to the increased awareness of the risks of childhood obesity.

risperidone they gained 11 pounds and with haldol, they gained 8 pounds. The most extreme weight gain was associated with clozapine in another study comparing clozapine and olanzapine. In a review of the use of antipsychotics in children, the increase in weight was: 4% for ziprazidone, 7% for clozapine, and 17% for risperidone. The two antipsychotics producing the least weight gain have been ziprazidone and aripiprazole. A study suggested that after an initial sharp increase, there is a weight plateau at about 2 months after which weight tends to remain stable.

Management relies on behavioral programs. Pharmacological interventions are unproven. No medication can be recommended for routine clinical use to lose weight. Weight gain with these drugs is now recognized as a significant problem and hopefully new strategies and new drugs will be developed to minimize this in the future.

Blood Sugar (Glycemic) Control

Several reports suggest a link between impaired glycemic control (high blood sugar—type 2 diabetes mellitus) and atypical antipsychotics. The mechanism for this is not clear but may possibly be through hyperinsulinemia, or impaired sensitivity to insulin, and/or some toxic effect on the pancreas which is where insulin is made. There may be a link between antipsychotics and type 2 diabetes mellitus through weight gain. There is concern that a drug-induced type 2 diabetes may develop at an early age. In adolescents treated with olanzapine, diabetic ketoacidosis has been reported.

Management requires regular blood monitoring for glucose levels.

Hyperlipidemia (increased blood fats including cholesterol and triglycerides)

Changes in blood lipids have been seen such as an increase in low-density lipoprotein LDL ("bad cholesterol"), decrease in high-density lipoprotein HDL ("good cholesterol"), hypercholesterolemia and hypertriglyceridemia. These changes have been reported mostly with olanzapine and clozapine.

Management:

- Early detection and intervention to control lipids.
- Diet—usually a low fat, low calorie diet.
- Lipid-lowering agents (e.g., statins).

Metabolic Syndrome

There is concern developing that some of the neuroleptics, particularly the atypical ones, can produce the so-called metabolic syndrome. This syndrome is defined as:

- Abdominal obesity. This is obesity where the primary place of fat deposition is in the abdomen and is characterized by a large waistline.
- Abnormal blood fats such as elevated triglycerides, LDL and low HDL.
- High blood pressure.
- Insulin resistance (impaired sensitivity to insulin) and compensatory hyperinsulinemia (which is inadequate to decrease blood glucose). This may ultimately lead to abnormal glucose levels and diabetes mellitus.
- Some also include a proinflammatory (increased inflammation) state and a prothrombotic state (elevated risk for blood clots) in the syndrome.
- All of these put the patient at risk for cardiovascular and other diseases.

Excess prolactin production may produce sexual dysfunction, delayed puberty, delayed growth, menstrual irregularities, gynecomastia (breast enlargement), lactation, decreased bone density, and increased blood prolactin level.

Hyperprolactinemia

Prolactin is the hormone responsible for milk production for breast feeding. Excess prolactin production may produce sexual dysfunction, delayed puberty, delayed growth, menstrual irregularities, gynecomastia (breast enlargement), lactation, decreased bone density, and increased blood prolactin level. These problems can be seen in males as well as females. In children taking antipsychotics, it is seen mostly with haloperidol, olanzapine, and risperidone.

Management:

- Reduction of the dose of the antipsychotic.
- Switch to another antipsychotic such as quetiapine, clozaril or ziprasidone.
- Use of dopamine agonists like bromocriptine (Parlodel) or amantadine (Symmetrel) to counter the effect.
- In nonsymptomatic hyperprolactinemia, treatment is controversial as a spontaneous normalization of the prolactin level has been seen in some children treated with risperidone at 1 year follow-up.

Cardiovascular Side Effects

Some changes in the electrical conduction in cardiac muscle may create the risk of arrythmias (abnormal heart rhythms). Such arrhythmias can be benign or dangerous. In children treated with clozapine, some had tachycardia (fast heart rate) in the supine (lying down) position with high blood pressure but none had serious arrythmias. In some patients treated with quetiapine some transient delays in the cardiac electric conduction were noticed which did not require intervention. The problem appears worse in adults than in children.

Management: Regular electrocardiogram (ECG) monitoring.

Anticholinergic Effects

This refers to various side effects such as blurred vision, dry eyes, dry mouth, constipation, and urinary retention or irregularity in the flow. More severe symptoms include disorientation, confusion, fever, and tachycardia.

Toxicity may occur if high doses are used, or if other drugs that have anticholinergic properties are also used. Examples of such drugs are certain antidepressants, diphenhydramine (an antihistamine), some asthma drugs (ipratropium bromide, oxitropium bromide, tiotropium), and others.

Management:

- For dry eyes: use of artificial tear drops medication.
- For dry mouth: sugar free gum or candy, oral lubricants such as OraCareD or MoiStir.
- For constipation: Use of a stool softener, increase in fluid and fiber intake.
- For urinary retention or irregularity of the urinary stream: consult the physician.

Clozapine—A Particular Situation

Clozapine has been reported to produce very serious side effects and its use should be carefully monitored.

- Agranulocytosis (no white blood cells) and Leukopenia (low number of white blood cells): There is a well-established risk for a fall in the number of granulocytes, which are white blood cells with a role in the immune response of the body against infections. Children may be more at risk than adult patients. Of 172 children, neutropenia (granulocytopenia) was reported in 13% and agranulocytosis in 0.6% over an 8-month period. Signs include sore throat, fever, mouth sores, and weakness. In spite of this risk, because of the severity of COS, clozapine may be the only effective treatment when all others have failed. Monitoring guidelines of WBC are very strict and must be followed more frequently in children and adolescents, females and certain ethnic groups like Ashkenazi Jews. Sometimes, even though a withdrawal of the clozapine due to the development of neutropenia had to be done, some children have been able to restart clozapine with intense monitoring in specialized settings.

- Seizures: These may occur in about 2% to 4% of the children taking clozapine. Up to 82% of patients on this drug exhibit EEG abnormalities (including non-specific abormalities). Anticonvulant medications have been used prophylactically when a child is a high risk or when high doses of clozapine are necessary.

- Hypersalivation (excess saliva production): This is common and its management can include the use of chewing gum, reducing the dose of clozapine or using anticholinergic medicines.

Clozapine should only be prescribed by physicians who are very familiar with its use and side effects.

48. If my child is to take medications, are there questions to ask the doctor?

- What are the brand and chemical/generic names of the drug? (Note that the chemical name may be the same as the generic name of the drug. However, this does not automatically mean that a **generic** version

---

Note that the chemical name may be the same as the generic name of the drug. However, this does not automatically mean that a generic version of the drug is available if the original drug is still on patent.

Generic

A drug identified by its chemical name rather than its brand name.

of the drug is available if the original drug is still on patent).

- How is it helpful? What is the success rate with this medication in childhood schizophrenia and in kids similar to my child—if this information is known?
- When does it start working?
- What are the side effects?
- Is it addictive?
- What is the daily dosage? How often should it be taken during the day?
- If my child misses a dose, what do I do? Use the regular dose? Double the next dose?
- What tests need to be done before starting the medicine? What tests need to be done while my child is still taking it?
- How will the doctor monitor the response and make changes in the dosage if they are needed?
- Which medications and what food should not be given with this medicine? Any problems with alcohol?
- Can my child take over the counter medicine with this medication?
- Any activities to be restricted because of this medicine? Like sports, protection from the sun while outdoors?
- How long will my child be on this medicine?
- What is next if this medicine is not well tolerated or does not work?
- What can I give my child if he has a headache or a virus or stomach pain?
- Is there a generic version available? Do the generics work as well as the branded versions and are they as safe?
- What is the cost difference between the generic and the brand?
- Where can I get a written list of the possible side effects?

- What are the long-term risks if my child needs to stay on this medicine for a very long time?
- Are there any very serious or life threatening risks, or any that will not go away if we stop the drug?
- What has happened in overdoses?
- What do I watch for about the suicide risk?
- Is it alright to get a 90-day supply or should we only keep a smaller amount on hand, like 15 or 30 days?

49. Are there any special precautions that we should take when our child is put on antipsychotic medications?

- Be proactive. Tell the doctor your experiences about what did and did not work. Do not miss the appointments with the doctor.
- Do all required tests as prescribed.
- Communicate any change that you, family members, teachers or others notice.
- Do not hesitate to call to speak with the doctor if something is unusual.
- Be sure the psychiatrist and the pediatrician or family doctor communicate with each other, particularly if the child is followed for another medical problem (e.g., asthma) and takes multiple medications. Be aware of drugs interactions, including over the counter drugs. Ask the pharmacist if you are not sure.
- Be aware of all the side effects that may be possible. Try to prevent some of them, like weight gain, by immediately putting a behavioral plan in place at home. With weight gain example, the plan might include reducing calories intake and increasing physical activities. Do not wait until it becomes a major issue.
- Protect your child from the sun with sun lotion to prevent hypersensitivity reactions due to sun exposure.

Be aware of all the side effects that may be possible. Try to prevent some of them, like the weight gain, by immediately putting a behavioral plan in place at home.

- These medications should be withdrawn gradually after prolonged use unless there is an emergency. Any withdrawal or dosage change should be done under medical care. Make sure you do not run out of medication or forget to give it. Make sure that your child swallows it!
- These medicines are not benign. Supervise your child when he or she takes them and put the bottle in a safe place when not in use.
- It is quite possible that your child's psychiatrist will use medications that are not approved by the **FDA** for COS but which have been used in adult schizophrenia and COS, in spite of not being approved. Just talk openly about it and about any concern that you might have. Many of those medications have been used for a very long time and there is a lot of clinical experience. More trials are on the way for use in COS. However, the lag time and doing research on medication in minors have always been a difficult issue. The FDA has put various regulations and incentives in place to encourage more clinical trials in children so we are hopeful more answers will be available.

FDA

The U.S. Food and Drug Administration (FDA) is an agency of the United States

50. How long should medication be taken?

Continuing the antipsychotic medication treatment is strongly recommended, as the vast majority of patients with schizophrenia will have a dramatic recurrence of their psychotic symptoms if they discontinue their medication. There is accumulating evidence that for each relapse a patient experiences, it becomes increasingly difficult to treat their illness and get them back into the more controlled state they were in before while on medication

There may be people with schizophrenia who do not need continued medication, but currently there is no

There is accumulating evidence that for each relapse a patient experiences, it becomes increasingly difficult to treat their illness and get them back into the more controlled state they were in before while on medication

way to accurately predict who they are. Medication discontinuation may be a consideration when the diagnosis is unclear or is complicated by the use of stimulants such as amphetamines, cocaine, or PCP. Almost all patients function better on antipsychotic medication. Additionally, there is accumulating evidence that early intervention is beneficial.

It is up to the physician, the child and you to discuss the duration of treatment as well as the dose and the side effects. As noted above, do not make any unilateral changes of medication without consulting the physician (including running out of medication for more than a day or two, as this is the same as "stopping the medicine").

51. What about long-acting medicines? Are they better?

The long-acting antipsychotic medicines involve injections that last for long periods and release drugs slowly. The treatments do not cure schizophrenia, but can help patients control their illness, with its delusional or disordered thinking and hallucinations, because the patients do not have to remember to take their medicine nearly as often.

Doctors and patients agree that one of the greatest benefits of long-acting medicines is often reduced side effects.

Doctors and patients agree that one of the greatest benefits of long-acting medicines is often reduced side effects. Pills produce chemical peaks and troughs in the body, as the level of medicine fluctuates around the optimal level. The peaks often tend to produce side effects.

In general, the effectiveness of the injections should be about the same as the oral medication, if taken regularly as prescribed.

The major risk of injectable, long-acting medications is that if side effects do occur, it can take weeks before medication leaves the body and the side effects resolve. In contrast, oral medication can be stopped immediately and the side effects often, but not always, resolve fairly quickly.

In Europe, 30% to 50% of patients with schizophrenia receive long-acting antipsychotic medication injections. By contrast, barely 5% of American patients have tried the injectable version of the typical antipsychotics, and they have mostly been desperate patients.

In the United States, the current available long-acting antipsychotic medications are Haldol Decanoate, Prolixine Decanoate, and Risperdal Consta. They are sometimes used in adolescents who prefer to get an injection every 2 or 4 weeks to control their symptoms.

52. I have heard that if someone is taking more than one drug there can be interactions between the drugs and they may cancel each other out or even hurt the patient. My child takes other drugs prescribed by our doctor. How can I check this to see if there is a problem?

Yes, it is correct that some drugs do interact with each other. This is a very complicated area since some drugs interact and prevent one or both of the drugs from working. Sometimes one drug increases the blood level of the other drug creating a type of overdose situation. Conversely, sometimes one drug decreases the blood level of the other drug producing inadequate effects. Sometimes

Drug interaction

A drug interaction exists when a substance affects the activity of a drug.

they interact and there is no effect at all. If three or more drugs are taken, this gets even more complicated.

Drug interactions will have been evaluated by the physician and pharmacist if the patient is taking more than one drug. It is important to be aware that combining medications of any kind, including over-the-counter ones, can produce interactions and side effects. This can complicate the treatment of COS.

All the medications that the child is taking should be reported to the psychiatrist and the pediatrician, including psychiatric medications, but also asthma medicines, antibiotics, over-the-counter cough medicines, antiacne medications, and all others (for example, certain "dietary supplements" such as for weight loss as they may contain drug-like substances). Your pharmacist can also help you. You should contact your doctor or pharmacist if a new drug, even over the counter ones, is needed, to see if it is okay. You may want to ask your doctor when he or she first prescribes the psychiatric drug what is okay if your child has a head cold, diarrhea, a fever or other common illnesses.

Following are some examples of possible drug interactions and your doctor should specifically clarify whether each drug combination is safe.

  antipsychotics and anticonvulsants

  antipsychotics and antidepressants

  antipsychotics and lithium

  antipsychotics and stimulants

  antipsychotics and oral contraceptives

antipsychotics and nicotine

antipsychotics and antibiotics

antipsychotics and blood thinners

antipsychotics and alcohol (technically a drug)

53. Why do we need long-term monitoring?

Long-term monitoring is important to reassess dosage needs, which usually depend on the stage of illness. Higher dosages may be required during the acute phase, with smaller dosages during residual or stable phase. The decision to lower the doses (which minimizes the side effects), or undergo medication-free trials, must be balanced by the potential increased risk for relapse. In general, first-episode children should receive some pharmacological treatment for 1 to 2 years after the initial episode, given the risk for relapse, before contemplating stopping the drug or even changing the dose if it is well tolerated.

In addition, continued monitoring is important to check side effects. Although side effects often occur when a drug is first started, they may occur at any time during therapy—months or even years later on a stable dose.

Some children may benefit from the use of adjunctive (add-on) agents, including antiparkinsonian agents, **mood stabilizers**, antidepressants, or **benzodiazepines**. These medications are used to address side effects of the antipsychotic agent or to alleviate associated symptoms (e.g., agitation, mood instability, explosive outbursts) which the antipsychotic may not control fully. Although commonly used, there are no studies that systematically address the use of these adjunctive agents in juveniles.

Some children may benefit from the use of adjunctive (add-on) agents, including antiparkinsonian agents, mood stabilizers, antidepressants, or benzodiazepines.

Mood stabilizers

A medication that helps mood swings.

Benzodiazepines

An antianxiety medication that raises the levels of gamma-amino-butyric in the brain.

54. What about comorbid (simultaneous) medical or psychiatric disorders? How is this handled?

Childhood-onset schizophrenia patients have a very high rate of comorbid conditions such as developmental problems and/or various psychiatric problems. For example:

- Conduct disorders.
- Learning disabilities.
- Mental retardation, autism, other pervasive development disorders, developmental language disorders. Note that the diagnosis of schizophrenia should be made only if the abnormal thought process does not reflect the communication impairment due to a language disorder.
- Autism. There is still controversy about the relationship between autism and childhood schizophrenia. Autism has its onset before the age of 3 years. It is currently presumed that autism does not protect a child from developing schizophrenia. "Childhood disintegrative disorder" resembles autism except that the onset occurs after 2 or more years of normal development. Also, children with developmental language disorders have been found to be at increased risk for psychosis.
- Children with Asperger's disorder lack the marked language disturbances associated with autism, but present with deficits in social relatedness (lack of emotional contacts, keeping to themselves) and communication (especially with social cues), and have a restricted (and possibly bizarre) range of interests. The lack of overt hallucinations and delusions distinguishes both of these conditions from schizophrenia.

- Substance abuse.
- Seizure disorder and other organic conditions.
- Attention deficit hyperactivity disorder (ADHD).
- Mood disorder. Affective or mood symptoms in schizophrenia should be brief. After remission of a schizophrenic episode, some patients experience a secondary depression which must be treated.
- **Obsessive compulsive disorder** (OCD).
- **Posttraumatic stress disorder** and child maltreatment.
- Suicidal behavior. Completed suicide and suicide attempts are tragically common in schizophrenia patients. The following specific factors further increase the risk for suicide in those with schizophrenia:
  - depression: especially if within 6 years of first hospitalization,
  - young age,
  - high IQ,
  - high premorbid achievement and aspirations,
  - awareness of loss of functioning,
  - command auditory hallucinations (hearing voices telling the child to kill himself), treatment non-adherence, and akathisia (feelings of restlessness) may also be related to suicide risk.

After remission of a schizophrenic episode, some patients experience a secondary depression which must be treated.

Obsessive compulsive disorder
An anxiety disorder with recurrent, uncontrollable obsessions or compulsions.

Posttraumatic stress disorder
An anxiety disorder that develops after exposure to a traumatic event.

55. What about birth control and pregnancy?

Schizophrenia may be somewhat different in girls than in boys. Girls usually have a later onset, they may have a different cluster of symptoms and the psychotic episode may resolve faster. Girls may require lower doses of antipsychotic medications to suppress the symptoms and may be more sensitive to the side effects from the medications. A possible explanation could be that **estrogens** may have a protective effect on

Estrogen
A female hormone that is produced in the female organs (ovaries).

However, when more than one individual within a family has schizophrenia, the age of onset seems to be similar for both sexes in the affected individuals.

the development of schizophrenia, though we don't know why. There is also the question of genetics influencing the sex differences. Clearly, the age of onset for girls is later than for boys. However, when more than one individual within a family has schizophrenia, the age of onset seems to be similar for both sexes in the affected individuals. It is not known whether or how the sex chromosomes might be involved.

Female adolescents with schizophrenia can use contraceptives. A few points need to be emphasized though:

- They are frequently noncompliant with oral contraceptives leading to unplanned pregnancies.
- Oral contraceptives may have drug–drug interactions with the antipsychotics.
- Long acting contraceptive medications may be the method of choice as this reduces compliance issues.
- It is not known if the estrogens augment the effects of the antipsychotics even though there have been studies suggesting it.

Adolescent girls who take antipsychotic medications may be less fertile due to the elevation of prolactin.

Adolescent girls who become pregnant need to be very carefully managed during the pregnancy and during the perinatal period.

- Neuroleptics increase the risk of congenital malformations during the first trimester of pregnancy. This may be less with high potency agents but one should presume the risk is real and take this into account in calculating the risks and benefits of treatment.

- There is an increased risk of preterm delivery and low birth weight infants.
- There is an increased risk of poor prenatal care due to the schizophrenic symptoms. Meticulous care and attention are required from the family and the support system.
- There is also an increased risk of unwanted pregnancies and reduced capacity to provide for the needs of the child due to the disease in the mother.
- The risk of postpartum psychiatric disorder is higher when there is a prior psychiatric history. Thus great attention after birth to the psychiatric symptoms is required. Delusions and command hallucinations must be monitored to prevent any harm to the patient or the baby.
- The risk of witholding medication for the psychotic process has to be balanced with the risk for the fetus and the patient. This may be a very complex decision requiring the involvement of the treating psychiatrist, obstetrician and family physician.
- It is recommended not to breast-feed the child as the breast milk contains neuroleptics (if the mother is being treated with them).

56. Should I get a second opinion from another psychiatrist if the diagnosis of schizophrenia is made or suggested?

Diagnosis is very difficult in children. Although the same diagnostic criteria are used as for adults, there are certain clinical features in children and adolescents that create dilemmas. A substantial number of children and adolescents initially diagnosed with schizophrenia may end up having other disorders when a clear diagnosis is able to be made. They may have bipolar disorder or **personality disorders**, for example. Moreover,

Personality disorders

A class of mental disorders characterized by rigid and ongoing patterns of feeling, thinking, and behavior.

the majority of patients referred to a national study of childhood schizophrenia did not have the disorder, but instead displayed a mixture of developmental delays, mood lability and subclinical psychotic symptoms.

There are several factors that can potentially lead to misdiagnosis.

- First, the relative rarity of the disorder results in a lack of familiarity with its clinical presentation.
- Second, at the time of onset, there is a significant overlap between presenting symptoms of schizophrenia and psychotic mood disorders, which are quite different diseases.
- Third, most children who have hallucinations are not schizophrenic and many do not have psychotic disorders.
- Distinguishing between the formal thought disorder of schizophrenia and that of developmental disorders (including speech and language disorders) can be difficult. Although most patients with EOS have significant pre-morbid abnormalities (behavioral problems, developmental delays, emotional instability), the presence of these characteristics is neither necessary nor sufficient to make the diagnosis. The vast majority of odd, developmentally delayed or language impaired children do not develop schizophrenia.
- Psychotic features such as hallucinations and delusions are required to be present to make the diagnosis. True psychotic symptoms must be differentiated from children's reports of psychotic-like phenomena due to idiosyncratic thinking and perceptions caused by developmental delays, exposure to traumatic events, and overactive imaginations.

- Clinician' biases may unwittingly influence diagnostic decision making. One study found that, in hospitalized adolescents, African-American youth were less likely to receive mood, anxiety or substance abuse diagnoses, but were more likely to be characterized as having either an organic or psychotic condition. Similarly, cultural or religious beliefs may be misinterpreted as possible psychotic symptoms when taken out of context.

- Cultural, developmental, and intellectual factors all need to be taken into account in the diagnostic assessment.

- Another issue is that patients often first present when they are acutely psychotic, and may have not yet had symptoms that meet the 6-month duration criterion. A tentative diagnosis must then be confirmed longitudinally. Some cases remit before 6 months, making it unclear whether they will eventually turn out to have schizophrenia. Furthermore, if the symptoms resolve with antipsychotic medications, the improvement may be due to either the treatment or to spontaneous remission. However, it is unusual for recovery in schizophrenia to be complete within 6 months, as negative symptoms such as lack of social interest or lack of motivation usually persist.

In terms of a second opinion:

If you are satisfied with the treatment team you have, if they are experienced and confident in their approach to the child's problem, then this should be sufficient—particularly if you see progress in the treatment.

If you have any doubts or issues, or if the case is particularly complex, you may want to consider another

If you are satisfied with the treatment team you have, if they are experienced and confident in their approach to the child's problem, then this should be sufficient— particularly if you see progress in the treatment.

opinion. In this case, it may be wise to head to a larger academic, medical school or tertiary center that has strong child and adolescent psychiatry services. As always this is a very individual and personal decision.

Psychologist

A mental health professional who provides assessment and therapy for mental and emotional disorders but who is not a physician.

If you have decided to get a second opinion, it is usually a good idea to discuss this with your child's physician.

Note the emphasis on the word "team" here. In many centers there will be involvement of not just a psychiatrist but other highly skilled and experienced medical professionals including **psychologists**, nurses, nurse practitioners, social workers, and others. The concurrence of the team in the diagnosis strengthens the likelihood the diagnosis is correct. If, on the other hand, you have only a single practitioner, particularly if the patient is a child and the psychiatrist is not a child psychiatrist, you may want to consider a second opinion.

If you have decided to get a second opinion, it is usually a good idea to discuss this with your child's physician. Although this may be delicate, a good and thorough physician will welcome a second opinion to validate his or her conclusions and to possibly add additional insight and experience. Your child's physician may even be able to recommend someone.

PART SIX

Treatment of Schizophrenia: Beyond Medications

What is Cognitive Behavioral Therapy (CBT)?

Is individual psychotherapy useful?

What about family therapy?

More . . .

57. What about Electroconvulsive Therapy (ECT)? Is there a role for this?

Electroconvulsive therapy (ECT) is a controversial treatment option that is rarely performed on children and adolescents for any diagnosis. There is a marked paucity of published data in this age group. ECT may be used in children and adolescents with EOS who are medication nonresponders, cannot tolerate medications (e.g., pregnancy), or a clinical presentation for which ECT may be particularly useful (e.g., catatonia). The clinician must balance the relative risks and benefits of ECT treatment, the morbidity of the disorder, the attitudes of the patient and family, and the availability of other treatment options.

Before an adolescent is considered for ECT, he/she must meet three criteria:

1. Diagnosis: Severe, persistent major depression or mania with or without psychotic features, schizoaffective disorder, or, less often, schizophrenia. ECT may also be used to treat catatonia and neuroleptic malignant syndrome. The diagnosis must be clear.

2. Severity of symptoms: The patient's symptoms must be severe, persistent, and significantly disabling. They may include life-threatening symptoms such as the refusal to eat or drink, severe suicidality, uncontrollable mania, and florid psychosis.

3. Lack of treatment response: Failure to respond to at least two adequate trials of appropriate medications accompanied by other appropriate treatments. Although there are no systematic studies of ECT use in adolescents with schizophrenia, controlled investigations in adults show that some schizophrenic episodes respond to ECT, especially when

Electroconvulsive therapy

A type of treatment, usually for depression, that gives a series of electrical shocks to regions of the brain, given in sessions that are separated by several days.

affective symptoms are prominent like depression or mania. ECT may be considered either when a patient is unable to tolerate neuroleptic medication at the therapeutic dose or when prominent affective symptoms or catatonia are present.

The initial decision to treat with ECT must be followed by a consultation with at least one other psychiatrist. The second psychiatrist should be experienced in the treatment of adolescents and ECT treatments.

Adolescents and parents should be fully informed about the procedure. Written consent of a parent or legal guardian must be obtained. Consent or assent of the adolescent should be obtained whenever possible. Some jurisdictions do not permit the use of ECT for youths under a specific age.

There are risks to ECT. Data is from adults as there is not much data from children. There are 2.9 to 4.5 deaths per 10,000 patients. Side effects are about 1 per 1,300 to 1,400 treatments and include spasm of the larynx, circulatory insufficiency, tooth damage, vertebral (spinal) compression fractures, seizures, peripheral nerve palsy, skin burns, and prolonged apnea (breathing stops). Again, keep in mind that this information is primarily from adults. See the website from the National Institute of Health for more on this subject: http://www.ncbi.nlm.nih.gov/books/bv.fcgi?rid=hstat 4.section. 1425.

Lobotomy
The surgical division of one or more brain tracts.

58. What about brain surgery for schizophrenia?

No brain surgery cures schizophrenia. There are two techniques that have been used. The first, **lobotomy**, is no longer done.

No brain surgery cures schizophrenia.

Lobotomy

In the past, before there were effective medications to treat schizophrenia, the surgical technique known as lobotomy was used to disconnect the frontal lobes of the brain from the rest of the brain. The frontal lobes are involved in the expression of personality and social interaction. These surgical procedures—performed mostly in the 1940s—were used to control agitated behaviors, or to treat distressing persistent symptoms. They are and were very controversial and are not used today.

Transcranial Brain Stimulation (TMS and TDCS)

The majority (about 75%) of patients with childhood onset schizophrenia still have impairing cognitive and psychotic symptoms after drug treatment optimization.

- Recent studies with transcranial magnetic stimulation (TMS) indicate moderate efficacy in symptom reduction in adult patients with schizophrenia. TMS is a noninvasive method to excite neurons in the brain. Weak electric currents are induced in the tissue by rapidly changing magnetic fields (electromagnetic induction).
- Transcranial direct current stimulation (TDCS) may be a safe and effective additional treatment of residual symptoms of schizophrenia in medication stable patients. The technique involves the application of very small electric currents on the skull. It is very different from ECT in that the strength of the electricity is much less. TDCS is not "stimulation" in the same sense as transcranial magnetic stimulation (TMS) or the stimulation of the brain and nerves with conventional electrical techniques. It does not cause nerve cells to fire on their own or muscle twitches associated with classical stimulation. It is

different from electroconvulsive therapy, which provokes a therapeutic epileptic seizure. The National Institute of Mental Health (NIMH) is currently doing clinical studies. It is still a research technique done only at specialized centers and cannot be recommended at this time outside of research studies.

59. What is Cognitive Behavioral Therapy (CBT)?

CBT is nondrug therapy that works by helping the patient understand thoughts and beliefs that are irrational, bizarre, or inappropriate. These thoughts and perceptions lead to negative reactions, emotions, and moods which are destructive to the patient. CBT attempts to break this chain of negativity by showing how these thoughts are inaccurate, distorted, and destructive. The attempt is to then replace them with useful, realistic, and helpful thoughts and then improved behaviors. It is very logical, concrete, and practical. CBT does not help the patients to understand why they behave the way they do but helps only to produce a change in the irrational behavior. The therapist will use and adapt techniques that are appropriate for the child's developmental age.

CBT is nondrug therapy that works by helping the patient understand thoughts and beliefs that are irrational, bizarre, or inappropriate.

CBT requires motivation on the part of the patient and the family, as the techniques learned during the therapy sessions must be used daily at home and integrated into the life and behavior of the child.

The techniques are safe and have no side effects. As noted, there are no medications used. However, they may take weeks or month to start showing results.

In schizophrenia, CBT is used only as an adjunct to medication when the child is stable and when some symptoms are not completely relieved by pharmacologic treatment. CBT is not always reimbursed by insurance plans for treatment in schizophrenia, however.

60. Is individual psychotherapy useful?

Individual psychotherapy may be very useful when the child is stable enough to accept the reality of the disease and to help deal with its long-term consequences. It will help with very practical issues like being compliant with the treatment, in particular the medications, learning to go through the complexities of daily activities and life transitions, and learning to socialize, and reach attainable goals.

Psychoeducational therapy will include ongoing education about the illness, treatment options, social skills training, relapse prevention, basic life skills training, and problem-solving skill strategies.

61. What about family therapy?

Families are in turmoil when one of their members has a serious mental illness. In the past, parents were blamed for the child's illness. Families need to be educated about the illness of the child, so that they can be more supportive and because they may need help with the management of schizophrenia in the home. Improving communication between all family members is helpful to the sick child who gets frequently confused.

Psychoeducational therapy for the family will increase the understanding of the illness, treatment options, and help developing strategies to cope with the symptoms of the patient.

PART SEVEN

Family, Friends,

and the Community

How do I deal with my child's brothers and sisters?

Should I try to get the rest of the family to help in the treatment of my child?

Does group therapy exist for schizophrenia?

More . . .

62. Do we still talk about the "schizophrenogenic mother"?

This is a concept that developed in American psychiatry some years ago in which it was hypothesized that the behavior of the mother (e.g., being cold, domineering, always placing her child in "double bind" situations etc.) played a role in the production of schizophrenia in the child.

This concept came from the analytic tradition of psychiatry which is one of several competing global concepts in psychiatry. This theory is not based on testable hypotheses and thus there is no clear way to prove it or disprove it.

The "blaming the mother" view has lost much favor because a more data-driven, science-based approach has become more predominant in psychiatry. A new viewpoint has been developed called *expressed emotion*. This suggests that in families where there was a lot of confrontational and emotional exchange and expression, the child would do worse than in a calmer family. It was felt that by altering the family environment, the progression of the schizophrenia (or other disease produced by such conflict) could be slowed down or even stopped. This led some therapists to develop techniques to lower or end highly expressed and charged emotion in order to improve the child.

This suggests that in families where there was a lot of confrontational and emotional exchange and expression, the child would do worse than in a calmer family.

Although the jury is still out on this theory, the advances in brain chemistry and the understanding of genetics and neurotransmitters suggest that the mother's behavior is not likely to be a primary cause of schizophrenia. Rather, it may be more a question of family (and not just the mother's behavior) environment influencing the symptoms, expression, and perhaps progression of the disease rather than actually "causing" it.

63. What is the role of family members and my child's friends in her treatment? What should we tell them?

Family members want to help their loved one. They will be willing to get educated about the disorder and to understand its causes and treatment. In some cases, family members may bring you new information, such as other cases in the family and how they responded to their treatments. Family members can help you to cope with your daughter's symptoms. You may also find that they will help you to communicate better with your child's therapist if it is difficult for you and they will be able to work as a team to support you.

Family members may be able to report to your daughter's therapist (with your consent) any symptoms that you might have overlooked or which do not occur in your presence. They may also help you out by occasionally relieving you of certain tasks such as helping with your child's homework or with the other children in the family.

Obviously, you must use discretion if you have certain family members who are not sympathetic, or are unwilling to help.

Several things to consider:

- Understand that COS is a disease and that your child is not responsible for the symptoms. Ask family members not to criticize or make negative comments but rather to be calm and supportive. Let them know that even if they try to be helpful, your daughter may not be willing to receive their help. They must try to be kind and patient and not take any of your child's comments personally.

Understand that COS is a disease and that your child is not responsible for the symptoms.

Support groups
A group of people with common problems who meet to share emotional support and practical advices.

Stigma
Literally a "mark"; something visible to others that sets an individual apart from others whether for justified or unjustified reasons.

You and your child have certain protections under law in regard to disclosure and discrimination. You may want to be judicious in what you say, and to whom.

Accommodation
A change that helps a person to overcome a disability.

- Manage expectations. Avoid expecting too much or too little and do not push too hard.
- Focus on the positive.
- Be alert to problems possibly due to the treatment.
- Do not attribute everything that goes wrong to COS. A bad day might be just a bad day.
- Treat your child normally when she recovers. Be alert to any sign of relapse. Encourage her to stick with the treatment and be honest and open with the psychiatrist and her therapist.
- Visit the therapist with your child if there is something you want to share or report. Make sure you set consistent limits and let your child know what is expected. Do not be too lenient because your daughter has an illness.
- Work with the school and the teachers as necessary.
- Do not hesitate to think about **support groups** for families.
- Take time for yourself to get refreshed so that you can better provide support later on.

64. What do I tell other people? There is still a stigma.

This is a good question because there is indeed a **stigma** around disease, particularly psychiatric disease. Several points:

- Not everybody needs to know. Not everybody needs to know everything. You and your child have certain protections under law in regard to disclosure and discrimination. You may want to be judicious in what you say, and to whom.
- One critical point is whether the schizophrenia is considered to be a disability. If it is, then there are certain protections and **accommodations** that employers

and schools must put in place. This subject is beyond the scope of this book but see the appendix for resources for further information.

• From the medical point of view, discrimination against people who suffer from schizophrenia poses barriers to recovery and successful adjustment at work, in the family, or at school. People with mental illness have reported that people they meet often have misconceptions about the risk of their becoming violent. Others blame them for not taking more responsibility in getting over their problems.

Families have formed public advocacy groups and have established networks to provide educational meetings, and lobbying. See the Appendix for further information.

You may want to speak to family and close friends who will be supportive and understanding as well as doctors and school administrators.

Again, not everyone needs to know, and you can be as selective about how much you disclose and to whom.

Be proactive about getting and giving information, such as books, articles, Internet links. Know that some people will be sympathetic and supportive, and some will not. It is important to you and your ill child that you both stay as positive and as hopeful as you can about the illness. More information is given in the Resource appendix.

65. How do I deal with my child's brothers and sisters?

The siblings of children who develop psychotic illnesses often feel guilty that in some way they have done something that has made their brother or sister ill. Disorders that affect the mind and brain are illnesses like any other. Brothers and sisters need to learn and understand why things have changed at home.

Childhood schizophrenia is not fair! It is not fair for the child with the disease and it is not fair for the family, in particular the brothers and the sisters. They may feel that their sibling gets away with things because of the illness and they are probably correct at times. Education about the disease and treatment will help them to understand and not blame the child with schizophrenia or their parents (or even themselves).

It is also hard to explain why one of the children has the illness and not the others. You should explain that there are interactions between genetics, biology, and environment that probably made this happen. Reassuring the other children that they will not catch it is important.

Reassuring the other children that they will not catch it is important.

It is also important to be aware of sibling interactions, to avoid any potential for violence and victimization. Living with a sibling who has schizophrenia can be very difficult. Brothers and sisters need at times their own space for their own healthy development.

If things get too difficult, you should consider family therapy or at the very least, a conversation with your child's psychiatrist and treatment team.

66. Should I try to get the rest of the family to help in the treatment of my child?

Yes, most definitely. Family involvement and support is crucial. The family needs to work as a team. Education of all family members is necessary as well as acceptance of the child as he or she is.

Structure

All children need structure and daily routine which makes them feel secure. Symptoms are more severe when there are life changes.

- Set clear rules and expectations for the child.
- Give the rules in a positive way. For example, "Do your homework before watching TV," instead of "No TV until your homework is done."
- Structure and schedule activities for each day, have family dinner, homework, and bedtime at the same time most days.
- If a change happens, help your child to accept it. Nobody likes change, least of all a child with schizophrenia.

Discipline

Misbehavior occurs and frequently has nothing to do with the illness.

- Set up a behavioral program for the child and reward good behavior with points or stickers. The rewards (and punishments) will depend on the age, **temperament**, and personality of each child. Have the child decide on which behavior he wants to work on. Give small rewards, not big or expensive items. Praise is a fine reward in many circumstances along with a little treat (such as some quality time, playing a game together, reading a special book, a special snack, or a token for a movie).
- Do not let the child with schizophrenia avoid taking responsibility for negative behavior that he or she can control.

Temperament

A person's inborn pattern of reacting to events.

Do not let the child with schizophrenia avoid taking responsibility for negative behavior that he or she can control.

Group therapy

Therapy where a group of people having similar emotional problems meet with a therapist to work on specific related treatment issues.

67. Does group therapy exist for schizophrenia?

Yes, these groups do exist. There are two types of groups. One is a support group and the other is an actual therapy group. The former may include both the children and parents, while the therapy groups are usually restricted to the affected children alone.

Support groups are very useful as they provide understanding and mutual acceptance. Children can develop a sense of camaraderie with others who have to struggle through the same difficulties. Helpful strategies are frequently discussed, about how to deal with symptoms, how to become more active, how to make friends, and how to get along better with people (social skills training).

A recent review of many studies has indicated that group therapy can be effective in 80% of the outpatient studies and 67% of the inpatient studies. Long-term groups were more effective than short-term groups and action oriented groups more effective than insight oriented groups. The optimal number of patients is between five and eight. The inpatient sessions met three to five times a week for about an hour and the outpatient groups met weekly for 60 to 90 minutes. There is some evidence that they result in decreased hospital admissions. Many of the studies reported 95% attendance, which suggests, at least in the eyes of the patients attending, that these are worthwhile.

PART EIGHT

Treatment Centers, Hospitalization, and Residential Facilities

What role do therapeutic residential facilities play?

What about after-school programs? Are they useful for continuity of care?

Our child has now stabilized, takes his medicine and is doing rather well. What further outpatient treatment do we need?

More . . .

68. What about hospitalization? When is it needed and when is voluntary hospitalization worthwhile? Should it be short-term or long-term?

Acute hospitalization for a child with schizophrenia will be necessary in case of danger to self or others, if the child is not functioning at home and/or other environments (school, social situations), if there are severe symptoms (severe delusions or hallucinations, refusal to eat, catatonia, agitation, refusal of treatment, inability to care for oneself), and in the complicated cases with other medical or psychiatric problems involved (e.g., depression, alcohol). In other words, all serious situations that may impair the child's development or where the home situation is no longer able to deal with the severe level of the problems.

The admission to the hospital or mental facility may be voluntary or involuntary, depending on the situation and the local laws.

The admission to the hospital or mental facility may be voluntary or involuntary, depending on the situation and the local laws. Short-term or long-term hospitalization will depend on the response of the child to the treatment but also on the availability of the local treatment resources and the ability of the family to provide treatment while the child is living in the home.

In many cases, the units are locked. Although the patients are usually free to walk around the unit (unless violent or severely ill) they cannot leave the unit without an escort and a pass.

Most people with schizophrenia will need to be hospitalized at one point in their life and you should check that your child's health insurance will cover this.

In general, the hospitalization should be only as long as needed to stabilize and treat the patient. The admission will allow for evaluation or reevaluation, review, and change (if needed) of medications; and restarting medications that might have been stopped but which are still necessary; as well as treating an acute issue such as catatonia, if that is what precipitated the admission. Other therapies such as cognitive behavioral therapy or group therapy can be started if they are available at that facility. Many feel that the structured nature of hospitalization (rigid meal times, medicine schedules, therapy sessions) also plays a very positive role in grounding the patient to reality. Some have called this *milieu therapy*. After discharge, some patients do well in step-down units such as therapeutic community residences before going home or day treatment programs, if the child is able to return home.

69. What role do therapeutic residential facilities play?

It is only when the child or adolescent cannot be maintained safely at home that residential treatment will be recommended. Usually, the child who needs such a facility has a severe illness, may have had multiple hospitalizations with outpatient treatment failures and staying at home presents too many risks for himself or the family. Often, the child has already been classified by the child-study team as having a mental illness and his treatment in such a restrictive facility has been approved by the treatment team.

As noted above, sometimes patients will go to a residential facility for a short length of time as a type of step down after acute hospitalization. This helps to smooth the way back into the home environment.

70. What about day treatment programs?

Day treatment or partial hospitalization programs exist in many institutions where there is an inpatient psychiatric

Day treatment or partial hospitalization programs exist in many institutions where there is an inpatient psychiatric unit.

unit. In these programs, the child is brought in each weekday (sometimes 5 days a week, sometimes fewer) for therapy that is similar to or even identical to the in-patient therapy. However, the child goes home at the end of each day, around 3 pm. Lunch is served and sometimes the day starts with breakfast. There are group meetings, individual meetings, and family sessions similar to those in inpatient units. There is usually a fairly large staff so that there can be individual interaction and treatment.

Sometimes these units are not locked as inpatient units are. That is, the unit may be locked from the outside preventing outsiders from getting in without permission but the door can be opened from the inside so that the staff and patients can freely walk out to other parts of the hospital. The length of stay can be from weeks to months depending upon the functionality and progress of the child.

These programs, with both educational and mental health services, are often recommended. Specific attention should be paid to the long-term needs of these children, with provision of vocational and independent life skills training.

71. What about after-school programs? Are they useful for continuity of care?

Therapeutic after-school programs are frequently a step down from a day program, as the child is still followed every day by the treatment team, and is provided structure and support. Contacts with the school and family meetings are necessary. Therapeutic after-school programs can be very useful on two fronts. First, they supervise and focus the child after school lets out and until the parents return from work. In addition to structure and supervision, these programs also provide formal therapy. This is the ideal continuity of care, especially if the child has been followed in the same community, from inpatient treatment to day program to after-school program, sometimes with the same team of professionals, including a case management program.

Nontherapeutic after-school programs may be useful later on as they provide structure, supervision, and recreation. They appear to be most useful for young children in grades 1 to 5. Not all school systems provide such programs. Sometimes churches, YMCAs, or other organizations run after school programs.

72. Our child has now stabilized, takes his medicine, and is doing rather well. What further outpatient treatment do we need?

This is the most frequent and happy situation—when the child is in a stable phase, has a supportive family, takes his medications regularly, and is able to attend school. Support systems in the community are quite helpful and help to take some of the burden off the family.

Examples of outpatient treatments less intensive than day or after-school treatment programs include:

- Group therapy to deal, for example, with anger control issues and poor social skills.
- Support groups to have contacts with other children sharing the same disease.
- Community management programs, which can be very useful in providing links to community agencies, like advocacy groups, legal support, and summer camps.
- In-home services, such as behavioral therapists coming to the home to work with the child and the family, and mentors.

- Individual therapy.
- Family therapy.
- Medication monitoring.

A growing interest among professionals is the concept of psychiatric rehabilitation, which provides the message that restoration and hope for a meaningful life, is possible by improving the social and vocational functions. Functional outcome may be more important than the full relief of symptoms like delusions and hallucinations. In this model, all the above therapies are combined to improve recovery. Many programs have been developed. For example:

- Assertive Community Treatment (ACT) or Program of Assertive Community Treatment (PACT) are intended to keep patients out of hospitals, providing treatment in the community, available 24 hours per day and 7 days per week.
- Some Model Rehabilitation Programs like:
  - Jump Start, which was developed for young adults aged 16 to 26 years to avoid gaps in the mental health system for those who aged out, was held on a college campus, using mentors assigned to the students to provide help to facilitate a normal life as well as helping with career goals and normal recreational activities. Unfortunately, it was discontinued due to lack of funding.
  - Some other programs like The Village in California (www.village-isa.org).
  - Vinfen in Southern New England (www.vinfen. org), a private, not-for-profit organization providing housing and services for people with psychiatric disabilities. See the resources in the Appendix.

Your child's doctor or counselor will help you to contact and obtain these services.

PART NINE

Surviving

How do we reduce the risks of relapse and decrease any residual symptoms?

What do I do if my daughter wants to stop taking her medications?

How do we help our child cope? Any particular strategies or pointers?

More . . .

73. What if we cannot afford the medications? Are we stuck? Is there any way to get help?

Many of the companies that manufacture the medications have assistance programs to provide either a discount or free medications for patients who cannot afford them.

Yes. Many of the companies that manufacture the medications have assistance programs to provide either a discount or free medications for patients who cannot afford them. The first places to look are RxHope and the Pharmaceutical Research and Manufacturers Association (PhRMA) websites. They support many of these special programs and have a website where you can check:

- RxHope, (https://www.rxhope.com/Patient/Home. aspx). Start on this page to identify the appropriate manufacturer or company for the drug you need. They have an extensive list with Internet links to individual pharmaceutical companies with patient assistance programs (www.rxhope.com/Patient/Company_ Links.aspx).
- The Partnership for Prescription Assistance at (www.pparx.org/Intro.php) for further information. They also publish a directory of programs for those who cannot afford the medicines. Your doctor can request this by calling 202-835-3450.
- NeedyMeds.com, a nonprofit information organization (www.needymeds.com).
- Partnership for Patient Assistance, sponsored by the Pharmaceutical Research and Manufacturers of America (PhRMA) (www.pparx.org/Intro.php).
- RxAssist (www.rxassist.org/) provides health care providers with information on accessing pharmaceutical manufacturers' patient assistance programs, and includes necessary forms and letters of application. Sponsored by AstraZeneca.

- See also the excellent listing of such programs at Mental Health Today: www.mental-health-today.com/medsassist.htm, where it lists specific programs:
  - Patient Assistance Programs Listed by Psychotropic Medication
  - Drug Discount Card Programs
  - State and Local Patient Assistance Programs
  - Patient Assistance Program Application Links

74. What about generic drugs. Are they okay? How about drugs from Internet pharmacies?

Broadly speaking, the Food and Drug Administration (FDA) has indicated that generic drugs that it has approved are safe and effective. Discuss this with your physician or pharmacist.

Internet drugs, however, are a different story, if you cannot be sure where they are from. It is very unwise to purchase one of the drugs for schizophrenia online and give it to your child without a physician examining your child and prescribing the drug. It is also unclear whether the drugs are counterfeit or real.

The FDA has stated:

"Patients who buy prescription drugs from websites operating outside the law are at increased risk of suffering life-threatening adverse events, such as side effects from inappropriately prescribed medications, dangerous drug interactions, contaminated drugs, and impure or unknown ingredients found in unapproved drugs."

"The Internet makes it easy for unscrupulous people to sell drugs to patients without these safeguards in place.

A website may appear to be associated with a legitimate pharmacy when in fact it is not. Websites that sell prescription drugs without a valid prescription deny consumers the protection provided by an examination conducted by a licensed practitioner."

If you wish to read FDA's complete review of this subject, look on FDA's website at: www.fda.gov/oc/buyonline/faqs.html.

75. I have concerns about the psychiatrist using psychotropic drugs "off-label." Should I accept this?

A very large number of children and adolescents take psychotropic drugs for very different mental disorders and many of them have benefited from these drugs. Most of these drugs have been developed for adults, have not been tested for pediatric use and have not been approved by the FDA for treatment of children.

More research is clearly needed but there has been, in the past, a reluctance to do experimental drug trials on children. The reasons for this are many and include the risk of harming the child, the inability to get informed consent from a child especially a young child, forcing a child to take medication, legal risks for the companies, and the need to hospitalize patients for some trials. This view has largely changed and FDA and other health agencies, particularly in Europe, are urging and creating incentives for companies and institutions to test medications in children. Of course, these trials will be held under tight supervision and control.

The National Institute of Health (NIH) now requires that children be a part of their clinical trials and there are several trials with pediatric testing going on. If a pharmaceutical company conducts pediatric studies, the FDA may offer an incentive by extending the patent of the drug by 6 months. Many drugs companies have responded and the FDA has approved aripiprazole (Abilify) and risperidone (Risperdal) for pediatric use in children older than 13 years.

Having said all of that, there are still many physicians who will prescribe drugs for children with schizophrenia and other psychiatric diseases for which there is no approval for use in children. The justification for this is largely two fold:

- First, although the FDA has not approved a drug for use in children, it does not mean that there has not been any research on the drug in children. Often, there is a large amount of published data on research in children. Usually this data comes from small studies, studies that may not have been rigorously done, studies that studied nontypical patients, etc. While this data may not be enough for FDA to approve the drug, there may still be enough information in the medical literature for the treating psychiatrist to use a particular drug for a particular disease in children. Note that there is the so-called drug lag in which it may take a significant amount of time (months to even years) for the FDA approval process to review the information before approving a new use. Many companies will also not pursue studies in children for commercial reasons, feeling that the studies are too costly, too long or too dangerous for the potential profit years down the road. This is unfortunate (to say the least) and is being addressed by the measures noted above to encourage studies.

The National Institute of Health (NIH) now requires that children be a part of their clinical trials and there are several trials with pediatric testing going on.

Surviving

- The treating physician may have extensive positive experience of his or her own in using a drug off-label and feel that the use is acceptable. In most jurisdictions, the physician may legally prescribe a drug for an unapproved use. In addition, in some major academic centers there may be experience using these drugs in children.

The bottom line here is that this is a very tough decision that needs to involve the parents, the physician, the child (if appropriate), and possibly others, including clergy and counselors. The benefits and risks must be weighed and a decision made. If the child is severely ill and has not responded to the usual and approved drugs, the team may feel the potential benefits outweigh the potential risks.

76. Should I place my child with schizophrenia in a clinical research treatment trial for a new drug?

This is both a philosophical question and a very personal family question. Progress with new techniques and medications will not occur without clinical testing as noted in the preceding question. This means exposing your child to a therapy for which there is little experience, which may or may not work, and which may or may not have side effects. Without such trials no new techniques will be developed. In general, however, the drug has already been tried and it has been found that the benefits outweigh the risks in adults and is probably approved for adults with schizophrenia. Thus, it is not as if the trial represents the first use of a new drug in human beings. Nevertheless, since children are clearly not small adults—they absorb, metabolize, excrete, and react to medications differently from adults and even other children depending on their age—great care must be taken and much thought given before deciding.

On the other hand, this is your child and the decision will have a large impact on your child and your family.

There is no correct answer to this question. If you seek such experimental therapies or if they are proposed to you, it is your obligation to fully inform yourself of the known data and to get an understanding of the known potential risks and benefits. Remember that, by law, you must be fully informed and enter into the trial freely and without coercion. You will be asked to sign an informed consent and you will be informed whom to contact for questions, issues, and emergencies. You have the right to withdraw your child from the trial at any time for any (or no) reason at all without prejudicing future care.

Research participants are frequently sought locally or nationally. Usually, the treatments are done in academic or regional centers that organize the trials and all treatments are free. Travel expenses may be reimbursed.

However, it is a commitment on your part to follow the treatment protocol put in place for the trial. You and your child's physician may review the ongoing clinical trials and whether your child might benefit from one of them. It is ultimately up to the clinical investigator at the trial site to make the decision if your child meets the inclusion criteria for the trial and if they can accept him or her into the trial.

Multiple factors must be taken into account, including how well your child is doing on the current therapy, what the trial is proposing in terms of drugs or other

It is ultimately up to the clinical investigator at the trial site to make the decision if your child meets the inclusion criteria for the trial and if they can accept him or her into the trial.

therapy, whether the proposed treatment is added on to the current treatment or replaces it, whether there is a period when your child cannot take any medications, the duration of the trial, what will happen when the trial ends (if the new drug has worked, will you be able to continue it "off protocol" under a special program?) and if two different treatments or drugs are offered, which one will your child get.

You can look for clinical trial at the worldwide registry website run by the U.S. National Institutes of Health (www.clinicaltrials.gov/ct2/home) and at the U.S. National Institute of Mental Health (www.nimh. nih.gov/health/trials).

77. How do we reduce the risks of relapse and decrease any residual symptoms?

There are several parts to this answer. First, there is benefit to early treatment.

- Studies have suggested that early treatment may lead to better clinical outcomes, while delaying treatment leads to worse outcomes.
- There was a much better outcome when medications were used than when patients received psychotherapy alone.
- The delusions and hallucinations were more severe the later the treatment was started after the beginning of the psychotic break.
- The longer a patient waited to receive treatment for a psychotic episode, the longer it took to get the illness into remission.

The longer a patient waited to receive treatment for a psychotic episode, the longer it took to get the illness into remission.

The bottom line is early treatment and regular medications.

Second, the medication should be increased (by the psychiatrist in consultation with the family and, where feasible, the patient) to the lowest dose that is effective with minimal side effects. The rule that "if some is good, more is better" does not always apply in drug therapy. One may reach an upper limit where effectiveness does not increase but side effects do. And, counterintuitively, some drugs will work less well at higher doses. The better the treatment is tolerated, the more willing the patient will be to comply with the medications.

Third, do not stop or change the medicine without consulting the treating psychiatrist. If new medicines are to be added on by another physician for another problem, make sure the treating psychiatrist is informed of the proposed new drug and decides if there is a significant risk for a drug–drug interaction (see question 52).

Do not stop or change the medicine without consulting the treating psychiatrist.

Fourth, do not skip doses. Make sure you check with the psychiatrist on what to do if a dose is missed by mistake. Whether you should double the next dose or just take the usual dose should be decided by the physician.

Fifth, do not alter the other modes of therapy (e.g., CBT, family therapy) without speaking to the psychiatrist and team, especially if the current mode of therapy is working. "If it ain't broken, don't fix it".

Sixth, where feasible, try to avoid major stresses and changes. Of course, things happen, but where possible, if one can predict a stress or change (e.g., graduation and new school, moving, new baby in the family, etc.) one can prepare for it. Speak with the treating team.

As you can see, once a stable state is arrived at, try to avoid changes and alterations in therapy and any stresses.

78. What do I do if my daughter wants to stop taking her medications?

If your child feels like stopping the treatment, discuss this with her doctor as soon as possible. As noted previously, an abrupt change in medication may precipitate a relapse, which will be harder to treat than the first or previous acute episode. Try to find out why your child wants to stop. Is it because of side effects with medication or perhaps because other kids are teasing her? Do not stop or adjust the medications on your own. This can be dangerous. Do not hesitate to ask questions of your child's doctor. Is there any alternative? Have your daughter participate in the discussion and the decision if appropriate.

Do not hesitate to ask questions of your child's doctor.

79. Is it appropriate to medicate preschoolers with these strong drugs?

An increasing number of very young children are taking psychotropic drugs. Deciding to give psychotropic medications to a very young child is always a very difficult decision in which the balance between benefits and risks has to be weighted.

If it is needed, the young child will be followed frequently in a therapeutic nursery and carefully monitored by professionals. At this point, little is known about the effects of the psychotropic medications on the young child's developing brain. Current theories suggest that brain growth may be modified by various environmental factors, including medications. This may be good or bad.

Antipsychotic medications have been very helpful in controlling aggression, hyperactivity, compulsive behaviors, and helping the children to be more receptive to other therapies and to learn new coping skills. Fortunately, schizophrenia is very rare in this age group.

Try to have treatment or at least an opinion from a tertiary or academic center where there is experience in medication and preschoolers.

80. What are the changes in the brain due to the antipsychotic medications that we know of?

The following are the structural brain changes that appear to be caused by antipsychotic drugs. Most of the studies have been done on rats.

- Increased size of the **striatum** has been found in human MRI studies of individuals taking antipsychotic drugs. It is not known whether this is due to the efficacy of the antipsychotic drugs or their side effects.

- Increased density of glial cells in the **prefrontal cortex** (nonneuronal cells that provide support and nutrition, and participate in signal transmission): which might be due to an adjustment in the neurotransmitters.

- Increased number of **synapses** (connections between neurons) and changes in their proportions and their properties, particularly in the caudate nucleus of the striatum. This may be secondary to the effects of the antipsychotic drug on dopamine or glutamate neurotransmitters. The changes may be due to the drug or be a marker for risks of side effects. This might help to provide an early marker for risk of

Striatum

Is a subcortical part of the brain. It is the major input station of the basal ganglia system.

Prefrontal cortex

The front part of the cerebral cortex, involved in complex thoughts, problem solving, and emotions.

Synapses

The gap between two cells.

tardive dyskinesia and indicate which individuals should not take these drugs.

The changes caused by antipsychotic drugs used to treat schizophrenia are similar in kind to structural brain changes caused by drugs used to treat other brain diseases. It is not yet clear what these changes mean and whether they have any practical clinical consequences. It is also problematic to extrapolate results in animals (particularly nonprimate species) to humans. So, it is not really correct to say that these brain changes are dangerous or that these drugs should not be used because of these changes.

81. What are the data for violence? Are schizophrenic children dangerous?

Most patients with schizophrenia (1% of the U.S. population) are not violent; however, violence is a problem in a small subgroup of the schizophrenic population. In a study of adult schizophrenic patients, 3.6% had engaged in serious violent behaviors and 15.5% had engaged in minor violence. By comparison, about 2% of the general population ostensibly without psychiatric illness engage in violent behavior.

Some schizo-phrenics with additional problems, such as alcohol or substance abuse, may pose higher risks for violence.

Some schizophrenics with additional problems, such as alcohol or substance abuse, may pose higher risks for violence. It may be necessary to include pharmacologic interventions for violence (sedative on an emergency basis, a change in the dosage of medications, or an adjunctive medicine) with other interventions, particularly with interventions for substance abuse.

In the stabilization and stable phases, persistent aggression can be associated with residual psychotic features, which should be one focus of clinical attention. More effective treatment will generally lower the association between a specific disorder such as schizophrenia and the probability of violence. Clozapine may have some specific benefit in persistent aggression.

There are other complicating factors in play here. Homelessness is a confounding factor. It is estimated that out of the 600,000 homeless people in the United States, 200,000 have either schizophrenia or bipolar disorder. These data refer primarily to adults. Although not all homeless people are by any means violent, there is a problem of violence in some cases, including homeless shelters. Many of these people are not under treatment, increasing the risk of problems.

It is generally felt that the major risk of violence is to the patient him or herself, not to others.

82. Can we predict violence?

Older studies have suggested that schizophrenic children and adolescents display aggressive or violent behavior before diagnosis could be made. Bender (1958) talked about "pseudopsychopathic schizophrenia" (a subtype of childhood schizophrenia) where adolescents developed antisocial acting-out behavior and were labeled "psychopathic," although the psychotic phase of childhood occurred later.

However, this view does not fully prevail anymore. Some data suggest that schizophrenics have higher levels of violence than the general population, but other data are less clear. Alcoholism is associated with a higher level of violence than schizophrenia. Conversely, other data show that 5-10% of indicted murderers have evidence of a schizophrenic (or other

Surviving

psychiatric) disorder. Interestingly, schizophrenics seem to be far more likely to be the victims of violence than the cause of violence. Most of this data are from adults.

Attempts have been made to try to predict which patients with schizophrenia would be more likely to be violent. Proposed risk factors include low IQ, a history of violence in the past, early onset, substance abuse, depression, conduct problems in childhood, having been physically or sexually victimized, and living in a nonsupportive environment, among others. However, in practice, it is quite hard to predict in individual cases.

On a more theoretical level, researchers found that the risks for violence are increased when the patient loses contact with reality, with the presence of delusions and hallucinations, when there is a flat facial expression and social withdrawal.

On a more theoretical level, researchers found that the risks for violence are increased when the patient loses contact with reality, with the presence of delusions and hallucinations, when there is a flat facial expression and social withdrawal.

83. What about crimes and schizophrenic adolescents in juvenile detention centers?

Over the last decade, the percentage of youths in jail and detention has risen in the United States. Youths with a mental illness are overrepresented in the juvenile justice system. A higher percentage of incarcerated youths have a mental illness in comparison to the non-incarcerated youths in jail or detention. Unfortunately, these mentally ill adolescents are often exposed to inconsistent psychiatric services.

A shortage of mental health services can cause youths who need treatment to remain incarcerated. Some detention center administrators report frustration with unnecessary incarceration. Without access to mental health treatment, these children are in jeopardy of continued, untreated illness, which may make it impossible for them to fulfill court sanctions or may lead to further criminal activity.

There are now many initiatives to address these needs. Working closely with judges, probation officers, defense attorneys and prosecutors, diversion programs like Assertive Community Treatment (ACT) accept court referred, mentally ill children and adolescents. It seems also that juvenile detention workers and judges are becoming more aware of these mentally ill adolescents and are referring them sooner to mental health facilities.

84. What about sexual offenders? Are they schizophrenics?

Sex offenders represent a heterogeneous group of individuals. Chronically mentally ill sex offenders present as a unique treatment challenging group. One study noted that 7% of sex offenders are schizophrenic and 2% are schizoaffective. Many also have a substance abuse or alcohol disorder, as well as other problems, including depression.

In some adult studies, schizophrenia plus a personality disorder (usually antisocial) or a substance abuse disorder was associated with an increased risk of any sexual offense and of physically aggressive sexual offenses. Only a very small minority of schizophrenics may become sex offenders, most often if there are other factors involved.

85. What about fire-setters? Are they schizophrenics?

In a study from Denmark from 2005, arson in adolescents was neither associated with previous admission to the hospital nor a predictor of schizophrenia even though 10% of adult violent arsonists in another study were reported to have schizophrenia or a delusional disorder.

Similar to the previous question about sexual offenders, there seems to be an increased number of schizophrenics among fire-setters but among schizophrenics, the number who are or who become fire-setters is very small.

86. How often do young schizophrenics commit suicide? How do we prevent suicide?

One in ten people suffering from schizophrenia commits suicide. Four in ten are known to have attempted it. Only 2% of those with schizophrenia who commit suicide do so in response to commanding auditory hallucinations.

There are some proposed suicide risk factors described in schizophrenia: male gender, high performance expectations, high educational achievement, chronic disease, worsening of the disease, death of a loved one, access to lethal weapons and toxic substances, and facing a crisis.

When a child talks about suicide, this needs to be taken seriously, as it is often a plea for help.

Attention to all aspects of the care of the patient is seen as critical to the prevention of attempted and completed suicide. Assessment of the risk of suicide during transitions (life transitions as well as changes like leaving a hospital setting to go back to the community) must be done in addition to any routine assessment.

When a child talks about suicide, this needs to be taken seriously, as it is often a plea for help.

Pharmacotherapy for these target symptoms requires optimal dosing, optimal duration of treatment, and

adherence. There is some evidence that second genera-
tion antipsychotics are more effective than first gener-
ation ones in the treatment of these symptoms. In the
face of persisting suicidal thoughts, clozapine has been
shown to be more effective than other antipsychotics.
Discuss this with your child's psychiatrist.

From 11-year-old Wang:

*I have been hearing two voices in my head for several
months now and they laugh at me and make fun of me.
They call me stupid and say that I am no good and should
not be here. For a long time I ignored them but now they
are louder and meaner and I really don't like this at all.
Last week I got very upset and sad about this and the
voices told me that was because I was so stupid and that I
did not deserve to live. I got very depressed about this but I
think they are right. I took some strong pills from my dad's
medicine cabinet that he uses to sleep after he comes back
from a business trip. I think if I take these pills and sleep
forever then the voices will not bother me anymore.*

87. What if my child needs restraints or seclusion in the hospital?

There are special restrictions about restraints and
seclusion in facilities for children. The use of restraints
and seclusion is limited to emergency situations to
protect the immediate physical safety of the person or
others. They can only be done by individuals trained
both in the physiological and psychological impact of
restraint and seclusion, and also in the monitoring of
physical signs of distress, and in the prevention of
restraint and seclusion use.

A supervisor or senior staff person, trained in restraint
and seclusion and competent to make a face-to-face

evaluation, should make a patient assessment within 1 hour of the initiation of restraint or seclusion, and continue to monitor the duration of its use. Time-out and physical escorts (being removed from a location due to agitation in order to be able to calm down) are not defined as seclusion or restraint. Mechanical restraints and sedating medications may only be used when a staff member is continuously monitoring face-to-face. This is always a medical decision within the legal and administrative framework in place.

88. Does my son need special education (special ed) because of his schizophrenia?

Cognitive and neurological deficits often mark the onset of schizophrenia. Changes in academic perform-ance may signal early difficulties and may continue to occur after the diagnosis is established.

Appropriate special education services are often a neces-sary component of a comprehensive treatment program. Children and adolescents with schizophrenia generally do not do well in standard classroom settings and often need a specialized classroom with low levels of stimula-tion, an individualized curriculum (**IEP** or individual-ized educational plan) that recognizes their potential cognitive impairments, and a teaching staff specifically trained to deal with emotionally disturbed youths.

In some cases it might be possible for your child to remain in a regular school if special accommodations are made to avoid stress and allow him to function. For example, permitting him to have a special, quiet place to complete his assignments or take a test may be very helpful. Another accommodation is priority registration where the child is allowed to pick his teachers and class times to minimize stress and fit best into his routine.

Cognitive and neurological deficits often mark the onset of schizophre-nia. Changes in academic performance may signal early difficul-ties and may continue to occur after the diagnosis is established.

Individualized educational plan (IEP)

An educational plan, written by the school (child study team or CST), for a student who qualifies for services under IDEA.

89. How should we handle the education of our son in each school?

The severity of your son's schizophrenia and the success of treatment will determine your approach. If symptoms are minimal and functioning is good, you may want to consider a regular school. It is worth discussing the situation with your son's psychiatrist as well as the school principal and the guidance counselor. Many schools have had experience with this and are able to give frank and clear advice on the situation.

If the determination is made to try the regular school, then see if any accommodations are necessary and feasible, and what the school is able to do. A discussion on the feasibility of special education, possibly in a different school specialized in this, should also be held.

Be sure to start this process well in advance of the school year since various meetings and discussions will be necessary, as well as the possibility that a referral to a psychiatrist designated by the school or board of education for evaluation will be required. All of this takes time and you do not want to do it after the term starts or on an urgent (and stressful) basis.

Pre-K and Elementary School

Schizophrenia can present in 6 to 12 year olds and even younger. Underperformance at school may be considered one of the first signs of vulnerability for schizophrenia. A very young child should be referred to a therapeutic nursery for assessment and treatment. Parents may ask for an assessment by the child study team later, while the child is in elementary school.

Schizophrenia can present in 6 to 12 year olds and even younger.

157

From 13-year-old Michael:

My parents took me to a doctor yesterday because they don't believe me. I am a flower and I can do a special flower dance and flower steps. They are very beautiful and I am happy to show these steps to everyone and maybe even go on television. I asked my teacher to let me show this to the class and she called my parents. I'm not sure why because these are very beautiful. I have to do these steps during sunny days because my ears turn to the sun to catch the light and give me energy to do the dance. My parents are very upset though I don't know why.

High-School

In a study, reviewing the high school records of adults with schizophrenia, and comparing them to a control group, fewer graduated, more enrolled in the general course of study than college preparation, more did poorly in English, social studies, and mathematics; more had an overall decline in their grade pattern, more had poorer attendance, and showed less interest in sports and dramatics.

College

Some people have to drop out of college because of their illness. They often wonder if they will ever be able to finish and get their degree. The answer may depend on the following:

- How severe the illness is
- How well the medicines are working
- How much support the patient has from family members and friends
- How well the patient is able to avoid relapses, by being an active participant in his or her own treatment (compliance with medications, involvement in

psychotherapy, insight in any change in feelings, ability to concentrate, ability to follow hygiene routine in terms of sleep, feeding, self-care)

If the child or adolescent had to stop his studies for a while but is planning to return to school, the family and student may have to make a few changes to keep the stress level low. Here are a few tips:

- To take one or at the most two classes at a time.
- To live at home instead of in the dormitory because it may be quieter and the student may be able to concentrate more easily.
- To consider switching to a smaller school where the classes are smaller.
- To choose a field of study that fits the academic and intellectual interests and level of the student, and is lower in stress than certain other fields (e.g., pre-law, pre-med).

If the child or adolescent had to stop his studies for a while but is planning to return to school, the family and student may have to make a few changes to keep the stress level low.

90. Are vocational careers and/or part-time jobs more appropriate than college or high school?

Vocational training programs or part-time jobs may be appropriate for some children or adolescents to address the cognitive and functional deficits associated with the illness.

Obviously, this will also relate to the interest level, skill set, and functional capacity of the student. If he or she is particularly interested in, say automobiles, it may be preferable to move towards a career as an auto mechanic, which can provide an excellent and enjoyable livelihood. One should also consider careers that avoid major contact with others. Using the preceding example, auto mechanics tend to work alone on a car with minimal contact with the public, compared to other service jobs that are highly interactive with others (and more stressful) such as office or retail-store work.

This topic should be discussed early with the school guidance counselors and administrators. It may even be worth seeing if the school's central or district office has more specialized services available to evaluate and then recommend possible career paths for a child with schizophrenia. Obviously, this is an area that should be discussed with the child but in a low-key, low-stress, nonthreatening, and nondramatic way over a long period of time. Do not wait for the last minute to start exploring this issue.

91. What do we do about friends and hobbies? And what about blogs and Facebook?

Schizophrenia can make it harder for an adolescent to communicate with his friends.

Schizophrenia can make it harder for an adolescent to communicate with his friends. Your child may have a hard time expressing his or her thoughts, and understanding what others are saying. He or she may not understand as well the subtle nonverbal social clues, gestures, dress, conduct, habits, interests, and the many other facets of social life that we take for granted and do automatically. Making a new friend may be especially hard. You will probably find that maintaining your schizophrenic child's social interactions and support system is harder and more labor intensive than with children without this diagnosis. But the harder work will pay off.

Work with your child, the psychiatrist and, if appropriate, the school to establish what level of information about the schizophrenia will be conveyed, if any. The school grapevine gossip can be very active, very efficient, and very wrong.

Encourage your child to:

- Develop a hobby and share it with other children.
- Help him or her to join a club (art, music, book club, etc.) either at school, church, social organization, scouts.
- Do volunteer work at the church or at an organization like the YMCA.
- Be open to friendships in school and help him or her nurture current friendships (home invitation to the kids, outings to the movies, etc.).
- Join a support group to meet others youngsters who have schizophrenia.
- Participate in a sport at school or the YMCA.
- Be very careful with what your child might put on social interaction sites and blogs such as Facebook and others. Try to see what content he is putting onto his site or downloading onto his iPod or MP3 player. Try to monitor your child's use of the Internet and see what sites he is going to and what chats he gets involved with. You may need to apply the parental filters in the operating system or provided by your Internet service provider to avoid dangerous or inappropriate sites. But be aware that there are public computers available, such as in the schools, libraries, and Internet cafes, where the filter levels may be minimal or do not exist at all.

92. What about dating? Should this be permitted? What do we need to know and do? Any issues with sex education counseling? Is there a relationship between schizophrenia and homosexuality?

Schizophrenia is a disease with serious disturbances in perceptions, motivations, and emotions. In a British study of adults with psychotic disorders, 82.5% of the men, and 38.5% of the women in this study were not in intimate relationships, whereas 42.5% of the men, and 38.5% of the women had never had a sexual relationship.

In the past, many psychoanalytic authors (Freud, Kempf) have said that paranoia and schizophrenia are one and the same disease, and that repressed homosexual tendencies and desires are the cause of paranoia. Others have said that severe bisexual conflict and confusion was the cause of schizophrenia. This is somewhat controversial at this point due to the switch away from psychological theories and more towards biological theories.

In terms of your child's wanting to date, this is clearly a function of his or her age and development. Although dating, intimate relationships, and sex tend to occur at an earlier age than in previous generations, each child is different and is ready at different times. This is an evaluation that is difficult to make in the best of circumstances and doubly so with schizophrenic children. Nonetheless, with the right person and situation, dating and relationships can be very successful and fulfilling.

Keep in mind that adolescence is a very tough transitional time for many people, whether schizophrenic or not!

Keep in mind that adolescence is a very tough transitional time for many people, whether schizophrenic or not! Support, counseling, nurturing, crisis management, intervention when needed, and all the other normal things that parents or guardians do will be needed here. Meeting new people and developing an intimate relationship can be very stressful, and having symptoms of schizophrenia can make things more difficult.

Many adolescents want to have an intimate relationship with someone they care about. It is important to determine (with the help of the treatment team) whether they are ready for it and to let them know that they may not be. They may find it easier and less stressful to focus on relationships with friends until the needed developmental level is attained. Practicing communication skills with friends will help in the future to better handle different points of view or disagreements that may arise in any intimate relationship.

Before dating, it is a good idea to decide whether to tell the person about the illness, and how to convey whatever information is meant to be communicated. Discussing these issues with the therapist first may help the adolescent feel more prepared to handle the beginning of a new relationship.

Discuss with your child important points for him or her to consider before embarking on dating and relationships. Tell him or her to:

- Try to determine if the other person is interested. No one, schizophrenic or not, likes rejection.
- Be prepared to deal with rejection when it does occur, which is never easy.
- Let a sexual relationship develop naturally from a caring, long-term friendship. Reinforce the need to practice safe sex by always using a condom, which will help protect against AIDS and other sexually transmitted diseases, and to prevent pregnancies by appropriate birth control. Good sex education here would be very wise.
- Not abuse any substances. This may be challenging but is definitely worth bringing up since certain substances such as alcohol and marijuana may worsen the symptoms of schizophrenia.

93. Is driving a car okay? Where we live a car is almost a necessity.

Many people with severe mental illnesses drive safely. There are, however, some mental illnesses for which extra precautions must be taken to ensure the safety of both the driver and other road users.

There are some data suggesting that schizophrenic drivers have double the number of accidents than non-schizophrenics possibly due to impaired cognitive and developmental issues. There are, however, no controlled studies on this.

There are some data suggesting that schizophrenic drivers have double the number of accidents than non-schizophrenics possibly due to impaired cognitive and developmental issues. There are, however, no controlled studies on this.

The issue of the medication being given to schizophrenics is interesting. Antipsychotic medications may impair the ability to drive due to drowsiness and other side effects which negatively affect the ability to pay attention and respond to things quickly. Patients who are prescribed psychotropic medication may be expected to have some impairment in general attention and concentration and in measures of psychological and motor performance. These impairments may be due to the illness itself, the medication, or the combination of both. Conversely, there is a limited amount of data that showed that patients on the atypical neuroleptics had less impairment than those patients on the older drugs (the typical ones). In addition, keep in mind that other drugs that the child might take (even over-the-counter drugs) may produce sedation and side effects which can impair driving. This can include sedating drugs like antihistamines, sleep and sedative products, and cold medicines.

As with all drug therapy, every patient responds differently and a judgment must be made as to whether driving by a particular child is acceptable. This will require assessment of the cognitive and developmental state of the child, the disease symptoms, control, and the drug(s) being used.

94. What do we know about prognosis?

Just as the symptoms of schizophrenia are diverse, so are its consequences. Different kinds of impairment affect each patient's life to varying degrees. Most will have an up and down course marked with some hospitalizations and some assistance from outside support sources.

Nevertheless, some generalities can be made:

- Children and adolescents having a higher level of functioning before the start of their illness typically have a better outcome. In general, better outcomes are associated with brief episodes of symptoms, followed by a return to normal functioning.
- Females have a better prognosis for higher functioning than males, as do patients with no apparent structural abnormalities of the brain.
- A poorer prognosis is indicated by a gradual or insidious onset, structural brain abnormalities, onset of the symptoms at an early age, negative symptoms at onset, and failure to return to prior levels of functioning after acute episodes.
- Adolescent schizophrenia is associated with a severe clinical course and seems to be worse than adolescent affective psychosis (bipolar disorder) and adult-onset schizophrenia. Be sure the diagnosis is as firm as it can be. It may sometimes require months or years to be sure.
- Symptoms and functioning may plateau after the first 2 or 3 years of illness without further progressive decline.

Surviving

- There is an extremely poor social outcome associated with adolescent schizophrenia. One study found that in adult life, 50% never established friendships or love relationships, compared to only 2% who had this poor outcome in patients with affective psychosis. About 21% never had a boyfriend or a girlfriend. Many subjects stayed dependent of their parents.
- At 10 years after the diagnosis, about 50% of people diagnosed with schizophrenia have fully recovered or made significant improvements and can function well in their lives. About 25% are improved but still need lots of support and 15% are not improved and need constant care and hospitalization.
- Up to 10% commit suicide.
- A history of schizophrenia in the immediate family or first degree relatives is a bad prognostic sign.
- Rapid treatment and response after the appearance of symptoms is of good prognostic. See the next question.

95. How is the outcome tied to the treatment?

Early treatment has improved the prognosis of the illness. Other important factors for a good outcome include:

- The relationship of the child and the family with the treatment team.
- The consistency of the treatment (do not skip medications, appointments, etc.).
- The different treatments involved (individual psychotherapy, medications, family therapy, multifamily groups, rehabilitation).
- The lack of substance abuse.
- Minimization of stressors.
- The rapid treatment of symptoms in relapses.

There is no clear evidence that one neuroleptic drug or group of drugs is better than others. Although there have been some studies suggesting the atypical drugs may be better than the older drugs, the data on this is still controversial. What is clear is that rapid drug treatment does improve symptoms and prognosis in many patients.

96. How do we help our child cope? Any particular strategies or pointers?

Leading a healthy lifestyle, reducing stress, and understanding the condition can help prevent relapse. Most of these points apply to everybody not just people with schizophrenia.

Leading a healthy lifestyle, reducing stress, and understanding the condition can help prevent relapse.

Exercise

Exercise causes the body to release endorphins which help one feel calm and happy. Exercise is also very helpful in reducing the risk of becoming overweight while the child is treated with antipsychotic medications (some of them produce weight gain).

Eating Well

Eating lots of fruits and vegetables is useful. A daily multivitamin may help cover the nutritional bases.

Avoiding Alcohol and Drugs

Many adolescents with schizophrenia try to find relief from their strong emotions by drinking alcohol or using drugs. Some even use these substances in place of their medication. This approach is very dangerous. Drugs and alcohol tend to make mood episodes worse, and quitting medication almost guarantees relapse. Substance abuse can be treated effectively. Obviously, this requires communication and an honest relationship with your child. As with all children, remember that kids learn much by copying. If the parents use or abuse alcohol and drugs themselves, admonitions to the child to not follow this behavior are often failures. Set a good example.

Developing a Daily Routine

Research suggests that a regular routine and sleep schedule can help schizophrenic children. This includes setting a reasonable and regular bedtime and sticking with it, getting up at the same time every day, with fairly regular mealtimes, homework times, TV times, etc.

Avoiding Stress

Help your child to avoid unnecessary pressure by setting reasonable goals. He or she may need not to take a full schedule of classes in school, particularly when symptoms are not in complete remission. See if there are ways to decrease stress at home as well as at school.

Creating a Relapse Action Plan

Know the precursors and early warning signs of a crisis: sleeplessness, ritualistic preoccupation with certain activities, being suspicious, unpredictable outbursts, being too quiet or isolated, changes in mood, bizarre behavior, and anything you know from experience that is an early sign in your child.

Take the Medications Regularly and Do Not Skip Doses

People with schizophrenia confuse real and imagined events. They might mistake remembering that they have to do something with remembering that they have actually done it.

People with schizophrenia confuse real and imagined events. They might mistake remembering that they have to do something with remembering that they have actually done it.

- Special plastic pill boxes that contain medications for the week, divided by day, with compartments for medications to be taken at breakfast, lunch, dinner, and bedtime can be easily and cheaply purchased in the drug store. Talk to your pharmacist.

- Make sure that your child is swallowing the medications given. You, as a parent are responsible for dispensing the medicine regularly.

Behaviors to Remember at Home
- Remember that you cannot reason with someone who has delusions.
- Do not express irritation or anger.
- Don't threaten.
- No weapons. No threat of physical punishment.
- Don't shout.
- Don't criticize.
- Don't argue.
- Don't bait the child into acting out threats.
- Don't stand over the child.
- Avoid direct, continuous eye contact or touching his or her person.
- Give the child an opportunity to feel somewhat in control.
- Don't block the doorway.
- Express understanding for what your child is going through.
- Speak quietly, firmly, and simply.

Steps to Be Taken If Symptoms Reappear: Depending on the Severity
- Call the doctor.
- Do not hesitate to call the police if there is potential for violence.
- Go to the nearest emergency room if there are critical symptoms.
- Contact family members or friends for help.
- Speak with your employer and the school so that they can support you and give you the time necessary for the medical appointments.
- Listen to the medical team.

97. How quickly should we act when symptoms appear, either the first time or after he has been diagnosed with schizophrenia? Is very early diagnosis and treatment a good thing?

There has been increasing interest in the treatment of first-episode psychosis (FEP) and in the early phase of schizophrenia. Antipsychotic pharmacotherapy should be started as soon as possible. One reason is that a delay in treatment is associated with distress, increased risk and worse prognosis. The second reason is that a longer duration of untreated psychosis (DUP), which is the time from the onset of the psychotic disorder to the onset of treatment, appears to lead to a less favorable outcome and a chronic illness course.

Antipsychotic pharmacotherapy should be started as soon as possible.

Many children who experience a first episode of psychosis can be treated at home if safety and support issues are well addressed. SGA medications are indicated in the treatment of a first episode of psychosis. Low, initial dosages of the medication should be used and titrated to prevent side effects early in treatment. This is important for later adherence to the medications.

The initial treatment response tends to be better in first-episode than in multiple-episode schizophrenia, but adherence to medication and treatment tends to be poor. It is important to maintain an active treatment relationship with frequent contact.

An important issue that arises for the patient with a first episode of psychosis is the duration of treatment (prophylaxis) to prevent relapse. A pragmatic rule of thumb recommendation to patients and their families is that children who have recovered and have been in remission on medication for at least 1 to 2 years may be considered candidates for a trial of tapering and stopping the medication. Withdrawal of antipsychotic medication should be done slowly over 6 to 12 months. The child must be monitored closely. Children who were ill for an extended period before initial treatment, who met criteria for the diagnosis of schizophrenia at first contact, and/or who have a history of violent or suicidal behavior may require more extended antipsychotic medication treatment. Without medication, 80% of patients with first-episode psychosis are at risk for a second episode within the first 3 to 5 years, and recovery from a second episode is slower and often less complete.

In terms of children who are already diagnosed with schizophrenia, rapid action is necessary if you think there is a relapse developing.

Determine if the situation is very acute or if it is a slowly increasing relapse. If acute, call your child's psychiatrist right away. If less acute, check when the next scheduled appointment is. Unless it is in the next few days, it would be wise to telephone the doctor's office and reschedule the appointment sooner.

Do not hesitate to call the police if there is a potential for violence or if violence has actually occurred.

If critical or urgent symptoms occur go to the nearest emergency room and tell them to contact your child's doctor.

Pay attention to suggestions of suicide or depression. If these are seen, act at once. Call your child's doctor or head to the nearest emergency room.

Pay attention to suggestions of suicide or depression. If these are seen, act at once. Call your child's doctor or head to the nearest emergency room.

Contact family members or friends to arrange your support system (e.g., caring for your other children, baby sitting, etc.).

Speak with your employer and your child's school and arrange time away from work or school as needed.

The rule of thumb here is clear: Don't wait. Act quickly.

98. Should a child or an adolescent at very high risk for schizophrenia be treated in the prodromal phase?

The prodromal phase of the illness is defined as the period of behavioral changes and symptoms that occur before the onset of clearly identifiable psychotic symptoms.

It is usually preceded by a pre-morbid phase during which there may be general deficits in social and school functioning. Not all behaviors and symptoms regarded as prodromal lead to psychosis.

We are better able to recognize the period immediately preceding the full onset of psychosis. This has been termed the ultra high-risk mental state

Nonpsychotic prodromal symptoms such as depression, anxiety, and social withdrawal are relatively common phenomena seen in different psychiatric disorders, especially among adolescents. These symptoms are not always useful or specific for predicting future psychosis.

We are better able to recognize the period immediately preceding the full onset of psychosis. This has been termed the *ultra, high-risk mental state*. It is defined by the onset of softer psychotic symptoms or brief intermittent psychotic symptoms lasting less than 7 days and a family history of schizophrenia along with a significant decline in functioning in the previous year. The ultra high-risk group has shown transition to psychosis at the rate of around 20% to 40% in the first year.

No definitive treatment can be recommended at this time for individuals meeting criteria for ultra high risk prior to the full onset of psychosis. However, there is some evidence that low-dosage risperidone or medium-dosage olanzapine may reduce the risk of conversion to psychosis. It is also known that delaying the treatment of psychosis is related to poor outcome. If this should occur, set up a consultation with a child psychiatrist.

99. May I force medications against my child's will? Should I go to court?

First, talk to your doctor and the treatment team. There may be certain legal and administrative issues in your area. Also, once a child is over the legal age he or she has legal protections and it may not be possible to force medication without legal intervention. We cannot give specific legal and administrative advice here. Below are some general comments but you must speak with your child's treatment team regarding your specific case.

Usually, young children do not refuse the medications, if they know that their parents agree on the treatment.

Adolescents with psychiatric disorders refuse medications for many reasons:

- A poor relationship with the psychiatric staff.
- Experience with or fear of side effects.
- Concurrent alcohol or drug abuse.
- Lack of awareness of the illness as they do not believe they are sick. This is called anosognosia.

- Delusional beliefs such as the fear of being poisoned.
- The cost of the medications.
- The lack of improvement.
- Confusion or depression.

Such patients may have to be medicated involuntarily. Studies suggest that the long-term effects of involuntary medication on individuals with schizophrenia are more positive than is commonly thought. The majority of patients retrospectively agreed that involuntary medication had been in their best interest.

These situations require written and witnessed informed consent, including rationale for treatment, potential risks, and benefits of the therapy for medical and drug treatment. If the psychotic state or the developmental level of the patient precludes this, or if therapy is refused, involuntary treatment involving the legal system may become necessary.

100. Does insurance usually cover the costs of schizophrenia treatment?

Mental-health advocacy groups have defined the idea of parity by urging that insurance plans provide the same level of benefits for mental-health care as they do for physical disorders and diseases. But there are many interpretations of what that means, and state laws run the gamut. In 1996, Congress passed the **Mental Health Parity** Act which was extended until 2003. Advocacy groups like the National Mental Health Association continue to urge Congress to pass legislation. The National Conference of State Legislatures offers a state-by-state breakdown of mental-health coverage laws.

Mental Health Parity

A policy that attempts to have health plans cover physical illnesses and mental illnesses in an equal way.

You will have also to contact your health insurance provider to check on your personal and children's benefits, as they vary a lot. A typical insurance plan will provide 30 days of inpatient psychiatric services if eligibility requirements dictated by the insurance company are met. The insurance company may not agree with the family or the doctor. There is usually a maximum of 60 days of inpatient services per year, with a lifetime benefit ranging from $100,000 to $1 million, with copay. Do not forget that **managed care** organizations function to keep medical costs down and will try to avoid hospitalization reimbursement as much as possible.

Children under 18 years of age who have disabilities might be eligible for Supplemental Security Income (SSI) payments. In most states, children who get SSI payments qualify for **Medicaid**. In many states, Medicaid comes automatically with SSI eligibility. In other states, you must sign up for it. And some children can get Medicaid coverage even if they do not qualify for SSI. Check with your local Social Security office, your state Medicaid agency, or your state or county social services office for more information.

The State Children's Health Insurance Program enables states to provide health insurance to children from working families with incomes too high to qualify for Medicaid, but too low to afford private health insurance. The program provides coverage for mental health services and is available in all 50 states and the District of Columbia. Your state Medicaid agency can provide more information about this program, or you can get more information at: www.cms.hhs.gov/home/schip.asp on the Internet or by calling: 1-877-543-7669 (1-877-KIDS-NOW).

A typical insurance plan will provide 30 days of inpatient psychiatric services if eligibility requirements dictated by the insurance company are met.

Surviving

Managed care

A system designed to control health care costs.

Medicaid

A public insurance program, paid by federal and state funds, to provide health and mental health care to low-income individuals.

Conclusion

In childhood onset schizophrenia, neurobiological alterations are seen before the onset of the illness (the premorbid phase) and may progress during the early stages of the illness (the prodromal phase). Further deterioration in brain structure and function may appear in some cases after characteristic symptoms of the illness begin (the psychotic phase), especially during the initial years. These observations suggest a critical window of opportunity, early in the illness, to affect lasting modifications in the course of overall illness.

A significant number of young patients are denied the most effective treatments because of the public's lack of education as well as that of the medical profession. A solution would be the development of specialized early-psychosis centers using a model of specialized treatment of cancer or pediatric intensive care. These rare centers exist already in Australia (Early Psychosis Prevention and Intervention Center: EPPIC), in Canada and the United States (see the resources in the Appendix).

Prenatal

The period between conception and birth.

Research is showing that a biologic or genetic predisposition (due to genes and/or **prenatal** or early childhood stresses) increases a person's predisposition towards thought and mood disorders. In other words, biology influences brain development (including the risk for mood and thought disorders), stress and trauma also impact the development of the brain, and possibly even gene expression. Increasingly, it seems, both biology (as a fundamental risk factor) and environment (as a contributing risk factor or triggering factor) are important in the development of mental illnesses.

For you, your child, and the family, schizophrenia can be a devastating disease that requires lifetime care, treatment, and vigilance. It can upset the family, produce issues with the other siblings, school, family, church, and so forth. It can be expensive and insurance may not cover all treatments. In summary, it can overwhelm your life. This is why you need to get involved with a child psychiatrist and treatment team to give you the support to survive the crunch over the long-term. As the statistics and clinical data show, the majority of the children who have this disease can do well and many even recover, but this does not happen on its own. Your active involvement is needed. Do not do this alone. Get your support in place too.

Resources

Recommended Books for Adolescents and Adults

The Complete Family Guide to Schizophrenia: Helping Your Loved One Get the Most Out of Life; Kim T. Mueser, PhD, and Susan Gingerich, MSW; The Guilford Press, 2006.

Surviving Schizophrenia: A Manual for Families, Patients, and Providers (5th Edition); E. Fuller Torrey; HarperCollins, 2006.

How to Live With a Mentally Ill Person: A Handbook of Day-to-Day Strategies; Christine Adamec; John Wiley & Sons, 1996.

I Am Not Sick, I Don't Need Help!—Helping the Seriously Mentally Ill Accept Treatment; Xavier Amador, Anna-Lica Johanson; Vida Press, 2006.

Brave New Brain: Conquering Mental Illness in the Era of the Genome; Nancy C. Andreasen; Oxford University Press, 2001.

Tell Me I'm Here; One Family's Experience of Schizophrenia; Anne Deveson; Penguin Books, 1991.

When Someone You Love Has a Mental Illness: A Handbook for Family, Friends, and Caregivers; Rebecca Woolis; Penguin, 2003.

In a Darkness; James Weschsler; Irvington Publishers, 1983.

Recommended Books on Mental Illness for Children

The following books are books written for children between the ages of approximately 7 to 13 years old who are trying to understand mental illness in their family.

Helicopter Man; Elizabeth Fensham; Bloomsbury USA Children's Books, 2005. For ages 9 to 12 years.

Sometimes My Mommy Gets Angry; Bebe Moore Campbell; Puffin Books, 2005. For ages 4 to 8 years.

Catch a Falling Star, the first book in the "Iris the Dragon" series for children with brain disorders. Available from the publisher's website: www.iristhedragon.com/about.html.

Edward the Crazy Man; Marie Day; Annick Press, Limited, 2002.

How to Be a Real Person (In Just One Day); Sally Warner; Random House, 2001. For grades 5-8.

Recommended Websites
National Institute of Mental Health (NIMH)

Child Psychiatry Branch of the National Institute of Mental Health
10 Center Drive, Building 10, Room 3N202
Bethesda, MD 20892-1600
Toll free: 1-888-254-3823
General NIMH website: www.nimh.nih.gov

Website on schizophrenia with multiple links on schizophrenia: www.nimh.nih.gov/health/topics/schizophrenia/index.shtml

Website for recruitment for NIMH studies: patientinfo.nimh.nih.gov/

Website for the NIMH publication on schizophrenia: www.nimh.nih.gov/health/publications/schizophrenia/summary.shtml

MedLine Plus: From the NIH's National Library of Medicine. General website with links to a medical dictionary, encyclopedia, physician finder, and more: http://medlineplus.gov/

Extensive links to resources and information on schizophrenia: www.nlm.nih.gov/medlineplus/schizophrenia.html

National Alliance for Research on Schizophrenia and Depression (NARSAD)

General website: www.NARSAD.org

Schizophrenia website: www.narsad.org/dc/schizophrenia/index.html

Schizophrenia.com—A nonprofit organization. Website with a lot of easy to read and practical information: www.schizophrenia.com

International Early Psychosis Association—Some listings of services available. Membership is free. www.iepa.org.au

NASCOS: North American Society for Childhood Onset Schizophrenia—Nonprofit organization with support for families and medical professionals

Home page: www.nascos.org

Living with Child Onset Schizophrenia (COS)—support for families: www.childhood-schizophrenia.org

Schizophrenia Society of Canada: Has a lot of information
P.O. Box 3528 M.I.P.
Markham, ON L3R 6G8
www.schizophrenia.ca

American Academy of Child and Adolescent Psychiatry:
General website: www.aacap.org
Child Psychiatrist Finder: www.aacap.org/cs/root/child_and_
adolescent_psychiatrist_finder/child_and_adolescent_
psychiatrist_finder

American Psychiatric Association (primarily for physicians)
1000 Wilson Boulevard
Suite 1825
Arlington, VA 22209
U.S. Toll free: 1-888-35-77924
1-703-907-7300
www.psych.org

The Experience of Schizophrenia. A personal story with a lot of information. www.Chovil.com

U.S. Department of Health and Human Services: Substance Abuse and Mental Health Services Administration (SAMHSA)

General website: www.samhsa.gov/SHIN/

Resources webpage: mentalhealth.samhsa.gov/

What Health—Extensive listing of links for health organizations: www.whathealth.com/organizations/

Support Groups

National Alliance for the Mentally Ill: NAMI
   Colonial Place Three
   2107 Wilson Boulevard, Suite 300
   Arlington, VA 22201
   1-703-524-7600
   General website: www.NAMI.org
   NAMI HelpLine: www.nami.org/Template.cfm?section=
   Helpline
   1-800-950-6264

SANE: The United Kingdom largest support group
   1st Floor Cityside House
   40 Adler Street
   London, E1 1EE England
   (In the U.K.) 44-020-7375-1002
   www.sane.org.uk

The National Mental Health Consumer Self Help Clearinghouse
   1211 Chestnut St., 11th Floor
   Philadelphia, PA 19107
   1-800-688-4226
   www.mhselfhelp.org

Recovery, Inc.: Sponsors self-help groups with a directory link on
   the website.
   802 North Dearborn Street
   Chicago, IL 60610
   1-312-337-5661
   www.recovery-inc.com/

ACTA: Assertive Community Treatment Association
   Suite 102 · 810 E. Grand River Avenue
   Brighton, MI 48116
   1-810-227-1859
   www.actassociation.org

Schizophrenia.com—Support group listing around the world:
   www.schizophrenia.com/coping.html

Information about the Brain

The Secret Life of the Brain—This site includes much of the
   content of the PBS television program called the *Secret Life of*

the Brain. The graphics for the action of dopamine and the anatomy of the brain are excellent. Also talks about the impact of drugs on the brain.
www.pbs.org/wnet/brain

Early Diagnosis and Treatment Centers for Psychosis and Schizophrenia

Website: www.schizophrenia.com/earlypsychosis.htm

- United States (15 Clinics)
- Global listings

Advocacy

Rethink: United Kingdom organization
    89 Albert Embankment
    London SE1 7TP England
    Website: www.rethink.org

Treatment Advocacy Center
    Website: www.TreatmentAdvocacyCenter.org

Bazelon Center for Mental Health Law
    1101 15th Street N.W., Suite 1212
    Washington, DC 20005
    1 202 467 5730
    www.bazelon.org

Schizophrenia-Help
    Website: www.schizophrenia-help.com/

National Dissemination Center for Children with Disabilities
    P.O. Box 1492
    Washington, DC 20013
    1 800 695 0285
    www.nichcy.org

National Mental Health Information Center (U.S. Government)
    Substance Abuse and Mental Health Services Administration
    P.O. Box 42557
    Washington, DC 20015
    1-800-789-2647
    www.mentalhealth.org

Appendix

Institute for Recovery and Community Integration
  1211 Chestnut Street,
  12th Floor
  Philadelphia, PA 19107
  1-215-751-1800 (ext. 265)
  www.mhasp.org/mhrecovery/index.html

National Empowerment Center (NEC), Inc.: Legal information,
  location of self-help groups, referral line.
  599 Canal Street
  Lawrence, MA 01841
  1-800-769-3728
  www.power2u.org

National Association of State Mental Health Directors: Gives a
  link to each state's Office of Mental Health.
  66 Canal Center Plaza, Suite 302
  Alexandria, VA 22314
  703-739-9333
  General website: www.nasmhpd.org
  Links to state mental health offices:
  www.nasmhpd.org/mental_health_resources.cfm

Professional References
American Psychiatric Association (2000). *Diagnostic and Statistical Manual of Mental Disorders*, 4th ed., text revision (DSM-IV-TR); Washington, DC: American Psychiatric Association Press.

Juvenile-Onset Schizophrenia: Assessment, Neurobiology, and Treatment; Robert L. Findling & S. Charles Schulz (Editors); The Johns Hopkins University Press, 2005.

Schizophrenia in Children and Adolescents; Helmut Remschmidt (Editor); Cambridge University Press, 2001.

MedlinePlus is a goldmine of good health information from the National Library of Medicine www.nlm.nih.gov/medlineplus/

Childhood Schizophrenia; Sheila Cantor; Guilford Press, 1988. Somewhat outdated now.

Handbook of Clinical Psychopharmacology for Therapists; John D. Preston, John H. O'Neal, Mary C. Talaga; New Harbinger Publications, 2008.

Clinical Handbook of Psychotropic Drugs; Kalyna Z.
   Bezchlibnyk-Butler, and J. Joel Jeffries (Editors); Hogrefe &
   Huber Publishing, 2007.

Help for Uninsured Patients
   See Question 73 for more information.

Partnership for Prescription Assistance
The Partnership for Prescription Assistance unites America's
   pharmaceutical companies, doctors, patient advocacy organizations, and civic groups to help low-income, uninsured patients
   get free or nearly free brand-name medicines.

   1-888-477-2669. Website: www.pparx.org

Clinical Trials
   www.ClinicalTrials.gov

   www.centerwatch.com/patient/studies/area17.html

Glossary

Accommodation: A change that helps a person to overcome a disability.

Acetylcholine (ACh): A neurotransmitter in both the peripheral nervous system (PNS) and central nervous system (CNS). In the PNS, acetylcholine activates muscles. In the central nervous system, ACh has a variety of effects as a neuromodulator, e.g., for plasticity and excitability. Other effects are arousal and reward.

Anticholinergic: An anticholinergic agent is a substance that blocks the neurotransmitter acetylcholine in the central and the peripheral nervous system.

Antidepressant: A medication used to treat depression.

Antipsychotic: Any medication that specifically suppresses the positive symptoms of hallucinations and delusions. This medication can also be useful in other conditions as a strong tranquilizer.

Attention-deficit hyperactivity disorder (ADHD): A disorder characterized by short attention span, hyperactivity, and impulsivity.

Atypical antipsychotic: One of the second-generation antipsychotic medications.

Basal ganglia: A group of neurons inside the brain that has an important role in the control of movements and behaviors.

Benzodiazepine: An antianxiety medication that raises the levels of gamma-amino-butyric acid in the brain.

Bipolar affective disorder: A psychiatric condition characterized by mood swings that occur episodically. Sometimes, particularly when very "high" (manic), people with bipolar disorder can have many of the characteristic positive symptoms of schizophrenia.

Catatonia: A condition characterized by extremes in behavior, of which the individual appears to be unaware. These behaviors include being mute or in a stupor and immobile. The other extreme is being in an excitatory state of an extreme frenzy or agitated excitement. This condition is not specific to schizophrenia; however, when it is periodically present in someone who has other characteristics of schizophrenia, it is then diagnosed as the subtype called *catatonic schizophrenia.*

Catatonic behavior: Behavior characterized by muscular tightness or rigidity and lack of response to the environment.

Cerebral cortex: The most superficial part of the brain, responsible for higher-level thought processes such as language and information processing.

Chromosome: A structure present in the nucleus of every cell of the body of any living thing containing genes. It is shaped like a long cylinder separated into two arms held together in the approximate middle by a structure called the centromere. The two arms have been named "p" and "q" arms, and the length of the cylinder has been quantified by the distance from the distal tip of the "p" arm. The "p" arm is usually the shorter of the two chromosome arms. People who view chromosomes under the microscope have noticed differences in the dark and light constitutions of the chromosome that may mean breaks where clusters of genes start and end. Thus, a method was developed for counting these bands. The band numbers begin from the centromere and go distally, using consecutively higher numbers on each arm. These two methods of measuring chromosomes and their size give geneticists the ability to know where different genes are located on the chromosome. Thus, when a gene is located on chromosome 6q21, 150 cM from pter this means it is on the sixth chromosome on the larger arm (the "q" arm) and within the 21st band down that arm. Its exact distance from the distal tip of the "p" arm is 150 centimorgans. More and more information given to the public will now talk in these terms, for example: "A gene for XX disease has been found by researchers on chromosome 6q21."

Cognition: The quality of the mind that allows animals to think, reason, and manipulate their environment to survive. Cognition can be measured by psychological tests. Of course, the tests are much simpler for nonhuman animals and are most complicated for humans. The well-known IQ is one measure of human cognition.

Cognitive behavioral therapy (CBT): This is a brief form of psychotherapy based on the principle that the way one thinks about something causes actions. Thus, it is focused on changing thinking patterns that lead to disruptive behavior. Several different techniques are available. This form of therapy is used to treat a variety of psychiatric disorders. Unlike the way it sounds, this is not a type of therapy that trains people to improve their cognition or intellectual abilities.

Command hallucinations: Imaginary voices that tell the hearer what to do.

Comorbidity: Coexistence of two or more disorders in the same individual.

Computed Tomography (CT): A form of X-ray able to view the brain in more detail than a standard skull X-ray. However, it has been largely replaced by MRI as a diagnostic technique to examine details of the brain. The advantage CT has over MRI is that it detects bone change, whereas MRI views the brain tissue, and is not sensitive to bone.

Conduct disorder: A disorder where there is a repetitive pattern of not conforming to rules and social norms.

Cortex (cerebral cortex): The outer portion of the brain. It consists mostly of the "gray matter" that contains nerve cells.

Delusion: A false belief based on faulty judgment about one's environment.

Depression: A major psychiatric condition characterized by profound sadness all day. It is usually accompanied by physical symptoms, such as loss of appetite, loss of sleep, and slowness in movements and speech. If the condition continues as long as two week without relief and interferes with a person's ability to function, it is then called major depression.

Disorganized speech: Speech may be illogical, not making sense, with an unusual choice of words or grammatical flow.

DNA: DNA is made of different nucleic acids: adenine, guanine, thiamine, and cytosine and is put together in the form of a triple helical structure. The variation in genes depends on the sequence of these nucleic acids in an individual's genes. DNA makes up the reproducing portion (i.e., genes) of chromosomes in animals and plants and makes up many viruses.

Dopamine: A chemical substance that is important for conveying messages between nerve cells in the brain.

Drug interaction: A drug interaction exists when a substance affects the activity of a drug, i.e., the effects are increased or decreased, or they produce a new effect that neither produces on its own. It can be a drug–drug interaction, a drug-food interaction, or a drug–herb interaction. Many drug interactions are due to alterations in drug metabolism.

DSM-IV: The diagnostic and statistical manual developed by leading clinical psychiatrists in the United States for the systematic evaluation of psychiatric patients and assigning diagnoses to groups of symptoms. There have been four major revisions of the DSM since its inception. It has two axes: It has 5 axes of which Axis I is for major diagnoses, and Axis II is for personality disorders.

Dyskinesia: Difficulty in performing voluntary movements.

Dystonia: A neurological movement disorder in which sustained muscle contractions cause twisting or abnormal postures. It may be inherited or caused by other factors such as physical trauma, infection, lead poisoning, or reaction to drugs.

Electroconvulsive therapy: A type of treatment, usually for depression, in which a series of electrical shocks to regions of the brain are given, in sessions separated by several days. The way it exerts its effects is unknown. However, it is usually not dangerous (though there are some risks) or painful and is accompanied by an anesthetic when administered. The only known side effect is memory loss subsequent to the treatment.

Electroencephalogram (EEG): Electrodes are placed on several areas of the head and recordings are made of the brain's electrical activity.

Estrogen: A female hormone produced in ovaries. It is produced in different amounts throughout the menstrual cycle and is reduced after menopause.

Extrapyramidal: The extrapyramidal system is a neural network located in the brain that is part of the motor system involved in the coordination of movement.

Family therapy: Any of several therapeutic approaches in which a family is treated as a whole.

FDA: The U.S. Food and Drug Administration (FDA) is an agency of the U.S. Department of Health and Human Services and is responsible for the safety regulation of most types of foods, dietary supplements, drugs, vaccines, biological medical products, blood products, medical devices, radiation-emitting devices, veterinary products, and cosmetics.

Functional MRI: A brain scan showing actions taking place in the brain in response to a stimulus. The stimulus could be anything, such as voluntary movement of the fingers to memorizing a set of words.

Gamma-amino-butyric acid (GABA): A neurotransmitter whose role is to inhibit the flow of nerve signals by blocking the release of other neurotransmitters. It has an important role in decreasing anxiety.

Gene: A functional unit of heredity that is in a fixed place in the structure of a chromosome.

Generic drug: Drug identified by its chemical name rather than its brand name.

Geneticist: A scientist who studies the inheritance of traits in humans, animals, or plants.

Glutamine/Glutamate: An amino acid that is a building block of proteins. It is also by itself a major neurotransmitter in the brain (i.e., transmits information from cell to cell); by stimulating the activity of the cells, it excites them into activity.

Gray matter: The brownish-gray nerve tissue of the brain and spinal cord that contains the nerve cells.

Group therapy: Therapy where a group of people having similar emotional problems meet with a therapist to work on specific related treatment issues.

Hallucinations: Experiencing something from any of the five senses that is not occurring in reality (e.g., hearing voices when no one is there to speak, seeing images of things that are not really there, smelling something that is not there, feeling something touch one's body when it is not actually there, or tasting something that one is not eating).

Homicide: The killing of one human being by another human being.

Ictal: Physiologic state or event such as a seizure, stroke, or headache. Post-ictal refers to the state shortly after the event. Inter-ictal refers to the period of time between seizure or convulsion in epilepsy.

Incidence: The term *incidence* of a disease refers to the annual diagnosis rate, or the number of new cases of that disease diagnosed each year.

Individualized educational plan (IEP): An educational plan, written by the school (child study team or CST), for a student who qualifies for services under IDEA (see Individuals with Disabilities Education Improvement Act of 2005).

Insanity: Mental malfunctioning or unsoundness of mind to produce lack of judgment and to the degree that the individual cannot determine right from wrong.

Learning disability: A disorder that impacts the ability to read, write, or do math and that affects a person's performance in school or in everyday situations.

Linkage: A relationship between two or more genes on the same chromosome that are relatively close together and the variations in the traits that each represents are inherited together in the same individual.

Lobotomy: The surgical division of one or more brain tracts. It is usually referred to as cutting nerves that run from the frontal lobe to the thalamus in the brain. It has been done in various ways, most often by inserting a needle above the nose in between the eyes. This serves to disconnect nerves connecting the frontal lobe of the brain to other structures.

Magnetic resonance imaging (MRI): A method to examine the tissue of the brain using a magnetic field and computer system. The machine itself consists of a horizontal tube inside of a giant magnet. The patient having an MRI scan lies on his or her back and slides into the tube on a special table. Once inside, the patient is scanned.

Managed care: A system designed to control health care costs.

Manic behavior: Feeling excessively elated and cheery with very fast speech and thoughts.

Medicaid: A public insurance program, paid by federal and state funds, to provide health and mental health care to low-income individuals.

Mental health parity: A policy that attempts to have health plans cover

Glossary

physical illnesses and mental illnesses in an equal way.

Microarray: An orderly arrangement of DNA samples to identify many genes at one time. They can contain thousands of genes on one small plate or "chip." An experiment with a single DNA chip or microarray can provide researchers information on thousands of genes simultaneously.

Monozygotic twins: Twins born at the same time who originate from the splitting of the same egg after it has been fertilized. The DNA is identical in both twins; thus the twins are sometimes referred to as identical.

Mood stabilizers: A medication that helps mood swings.

Negative symptoms: Those characteristics of psychiatric illness that present as withdrawn behavior, an expressionless face, a lack of initiative, a lack of interest, slow speech, not saying much when talking, slowed thoughts, and slowed movements. Sometimes these symptoms are confused with either depression or side effects of medication.

Neurodevelopmental: Happening during the growth and formation of different structures of the brain.

Neuroleptic: Any medication that when given to animals will cause catalepsy. This name then was used to label all drugs that had an effect on reducing the symptoms of schizophrenia. They are sometimes known as the "major tranquilizers."

Neuroleptic malignant syndrome: A severe, although rare, side effect of neuroleptic treatment whose cause is unknown. Some of the warning signs are fast heart beat, high fluctuating blood pressure, tremors, sweating, and fever. Cessation of neuroleptic therapy is the only treatment. This is a serious medical emergency that requires immediate treatment.

Neurons: A cell in the brain or nervous system that is specialized in sending, receiving or processing information.

Neurotransmitter: A chemical which is a messenger within the brain.

Norepinephrine: A neurotransmitter that regulates arousal, sleep, blood pressure, and may produce anxiety.

Obsessive-compulsive disorder: An anxiety disorder with recurrent, uncontrollable obsessions or compulsions.

Paranoid: Having excessive or irrational suspicion or distrust of others.

Personality disorder: A class of mental disorders characterized by rigid and ongoing patterns of feeling, thinking, and behavior.

Pervasive developmental disorders: Refers to a group of five disorders characterized by delays in the development of multiple basic functions including socialization and communication. The pervasive developmental disorders are: *Autism,* the most commonly known, *Rett syndrome, Childhood disintegrative disorder, Asperger syndrome,* and *Pervasive developmental disorder not otherwise specified* (PDD-NOS), which includes atypical autism.

Pharmacotherapy: Treatment of disease through the use of drugs.

Pituitary gland: A small gland at the base of the brain. Its hormones control other glands and have a role in growth, metabolism, and reproduction.

Positive symptoms: Considered the active symptoms of hallucinations and delusions of schizophrenia.

Posttraumatic disorder: An anxiety disorder that develops after an exposure to a traumatic event. Symptoms are re-experiencing the trauma, avoidance, emotional numbing, and arousal.

Prefrontal cortex: The front part of the cerebral cortex, involved in complex thoughts, problem solving, emotions.

Premorbid: The time period before any symptoms of a disorder, including subtle signs, have developed.

Prenatal: The period between conception and birth.

Prevalence: Prevalence of a disease usually refers to the estimated population of people who are living with that disease at any given time.

Prodromal: An early or premonitory symptom of a disease. If true specific prodromal symptoms are known, one can detect the illness early. These symptoms signify that the disease will be almost certain.

Prognosis: Prediction of how a patient will progress.

Psychiatrist: A medical doctor, specializing in the diagnosis and treatment of mental illnesses and emotional problems.

Psychologist: A mental health professional who provides assessment and therapy for mental and emotional disorders but who is not a physician.

Psychotherapy: The treatment of mental or emotional problems by psychological means.

Psychotic: People are considered psychotic if they have lost touch with reality, have delusions (i.e., false beliefs), and hallucinations. They often are exhibiting bizarre and risky behavior and do not seem to be aware that they are doing anything unusual.

Receptor: A molecule that recognizes a specific chemical. When a chemical message is sent from one cell to another, the chemical is received by a matching receptor situated at the surface of the receiving cell.

Relapse: Occurs when a person is affected again by a condition that affected them in the past.

Remission: The state of absence of disease activity in patients with a chronic illness, with the possibility of return of disease activity.

Residual: Having some nonspecific symptoms (usually negative symptoms), but no longer active psychotic ones.

Risk factor: A characteristic that increases a person's likelihood of developing a disorder.

Schizoaffective: Having both prominent symptoms of schizophrenia and depression and/or mania that overlap with the schizophrenia-like symptoms. However, they do not always coincide, so that sometimes the patients have only schizophrenia-like symptoms and at other times, although less so, only mania or depressive symptoms.

Schizophrenia: Any of a group of psychotic disorders usually characterized by withdrawal from reality, illogical patterns of thinking, delusions, and hallucinations, and accompanied in varying degrees by other emotional, behavioral, or intellectual disturbances. Schizophrenia is associated with dopamine imbalances in the brain and defects of the frontal lobe and is caused by genetic, other biological, and psychosocial factors.

Schizophreniform: Having the symptoms of schizophrenia, but too early in the course of illness to tell whether the symptoms are of a schizophrenia illness.

Serotonin: A hormone found in the brain, platelets, digestive tract, and pineal gland. It acts both as a neurotransmitter (a substance that nerves use to send messages to one another) and a vasoconstrictor (a substance that causes blood vessels to narrow). A lack of serotonin in the brain is thought to be a cause of depression and anxiety.

Side effect: An unintended effect of a drug.

Stigma: Literally a "mark"; something visible to others that sets an individual apart from others, whether for justified or unjustified reasons.

Striatum: A subcortical part of the brain. It is the major input station of the basal ganglia system. Anatomically, the striatum is the caudate nucleus and the putamen. It is best known for its role in the modulation of movements but is also involved in a variety of other cognitive processes.

Substance abuse: The continued use of alcohol and or other drugs despite negative consequences like social, legal, and relational problems.

Suicide: The act of causing ones own death.

Support group: A group of people with common problems who meet to share emotional support and practical advice.

Synapse: The gap between two cells.

Temperament: A person's inborn pattern of reacting to events.

Thalamus: A brain structure that relays incoming sensory information.

Tranquilizer: Any drug that is used to calm or pacify an anxious and/or agitated person. There are minor and major classes of tranquilizers which have different chemical properties and are indicated for different psychiatric conditions. The minor ones are used for anxiety in a person who has not lost a sense of reality but who needs calming. Major tranquilizers are the class of drugs used for psychotic symptoms.

Transporter: A molecule that carries a chemical messenger, called neurotransmitter, back to the cell that originally sent the message.

Ventricles: The spaces throughout the brain that provide a system for the circulation of cerebrospinal fluid. The ventricles in the brain consist of the lateral ventricles, third, and fourth ventricles. They connect to the spinal column and bathe the spinal cord.

White matter: Whitish brain and spinal cord tissue composed mostly of nerve fibers and its shiny protective coat called myelin.

Working memory: A more contemporary term for short-term memory. It is thought of as an active system for temporarily storing and manipulating information needed for conducting complex tasks such as learning, reasoning, and comprehending things. There are two components of working memory: storage and central executive functions. The two storage systems within working memory are for temporary storage of verbal and visual information. The central executive function is thought to be a process that is very active and responsible for the selection, initiation, and termination of processing the storing and retrieving of memories.

INDEX

Index